# A WAY TO NATURAL CHILDBIRTH

# MARIA EBNER
M.C.S.P., Dip. T.P.

Diploma in Physical Education (Vienna University) Former
Principal of School and Department of Physiotherapy of the
United Leeds Hospitals

# *A Way to Natural Childbirth*

A MANUAL FOR PHYSIOTHERAPISTS
AND PARENTS-TO-BE

By HELEN HEARDMAN

REVISED AND RE-EDITED BY MARIA EBNER

THIRD EDITION

CHURCHILL LIVINGSTONE
EDINBURGH AND LONDON 1973

## CHURCHILL LIVINGSTONE

Medical Division of Longman Group Limited

Represented in the United States of America by
Longman Inc., New York, and by associated companies,
branches and representatives throughout the world.

| | |
|---|---|
| *First Edition* | *1948* |
| *Reprinted* | *1949* |
| *Reprinted* | *1950* |
| *Reprinted* | *1951* |
| *Reprinted* | *1952* |
| *Reprinted* | *1954* |
| *Reprinted* | *1956* |
| *Reprinted* | *1958* |
| *Revised Reprint* | *1961* |
| *Reprinted* | *1964* |
| *Second Edition* | *1970* |
| *Third Edition* | *1973* |

**ISBN 0 443 01061 7**

Library of Congress Catalog Card Number 73 - 85388

*Printed in Great Britain*

# Foreword to First Edition

Nothing has been more remarkable in the practice of obstetrics within the last ten years than the increasing appreciation of the value of the principles enunciated by Edmund Jacobson in 1929 in his book, 'Progressive Relaxation,' and afterwards applied to midwifery by Grantly Dick Read in his two books, 'Natural Childbirth' and 'Revelation of Childbirth'. That being so, it was inevitable that some such manual as that of Mrs Heardman should be written. For it fulfils the important purpose of making available to those responsible for the care of the expectant mother detailed information regarding the methods by which she may be trained in the practice of relaxation in labour. So far as I am aware, no other book does this so well. This is partly because the author has had the advantage of having herself experienced more than once the sensations, painful and pleasurable, which in greater or less degree accompany pregnancy and parturition, and partly because of her long experience as a teacher of the art in antenatal clinics and labour wards. As will be seen by readers of this book, she does not rest content with preparing expectant mothers for labour but, with the cooperation of the labour ward staffs, stays with her patients throughout their adventure, seeing that they 'do their stuff,' thus, incidentally, being in a position to criticise her own teaching and assess its value as a help in preventing unnecessary pain and discomfort.

Of one thing there can be no doubt: the women who record their experiences in the letters from which the extracts published in Chapter VII are taken are remarkably unanimous about the value of the method. That being so, no one responsible for the care of the women in labour can any longer afford to ignore this new teaching. That is why I am sure this manual should be on the bookshelf of every obstetric surgeon and every midwife.

F. J. BROWNE,

1948                    M.D., D.Sc., F.R.C.S.E., F.R.C.O.

# Preface to Second Edition

IT was with interest and gratitude that I received an invitation from the Publishers suggesting that I might revise the third of Mrs Helen Heardman's original books on preparation for childbirth. Before finally deciding, I read again carefully the orginal text of *A Way to Natural Childbirth* written in 1948 by Mrs Heardman and was gratified to notice how much of the contents was still valid. Having worked for many years with her, I realised that methods of approach may slightly change but Mrs Heardman's pioneering efforts to give mental and physical help to the expectant mother were founded on sound principles. The work of the last eight years has helped to clarify some points, others are still debatable and will need clarification through future research. The Swedish remedial exercise approach has been replaced by an approach on a more physiological basis and the formal execution of exercises has given way to a more personal adaption of exercises to individual needs. Slightly more emphasis has been placed on mental and emotional preparation. The approach to the postnatal period has been brought into line with current practice which permits the young mother to get up much earlier. Provided the young mother is healthy and everything procedes normally, she is helped to prepare herself for a normal physiological function, which entails hard work and should therefore be preceded by a period of preparation and training in order to avoid unnecessary physical and mental trauma.

It is hoped that the present edition will continue to help the pregnant woman to avoid unecessary discomfort during pregnancy, approach labour with a comprehensive under-standing of the events which will take place and effectively and quickly recover afterwards to full health, ready to enjoy new responsibilities. It is also hoped that it will help her to participate actively during all the events of the childbearing cycle.

I should like to take this opportunity to thank the continually increasing number of medical men who take an active interest in this work. It is this interest which enables midwives, health visitors and physiotherapists to increase their knowledge and make this preparatory work scientifically sound and more effective.

As usual the publishers have continued to give never-failing help with patience and tolerance.

1970                                                                      M.E.

# Preface to Third Edition

It was gratifying to receive an invitation by the Publishers to revise the second edition of Mrs Heardman's original book. I had last revised and re-edited the original book in 1970. The fact that a new edition had become necessary in such a comparatively short time has proved that the contents of this little book has proved helpful to many expectant mothers and to many who are concerned with her future welfare. Those of us who have been concerned with this work can still be satisfied that we are working on sound principles. The altered approach of the last edition, stressing a more physiological basis, has been rewarding. Social conditions are however continuously changing and bring with them very often new problems. It is therefore important that all members of the team attending the young woman who is expecting a baby, try to give help to the solution of these problems, where it is possible. A small book of this kind can only hint at these problems. Fortunately many members of the obstetric team are well qualified to attend to these problems and give help wherever this is found desirable.

It is therefore hoped that the present edition will continue to help the pregnant woman to cope more easily with the physiological, emotional and social problems of her pregnancy.

I should like to take this opportunity to thank particularly many members of Local Authorities Health Services who have become aware of the problems of the expectant mother. New training facilities for all members of the obstetric team are made available and readily accepted. The Community can only be grateful for this positive approach to a true Health Service.

My gratitude is also due to the Publishers who have given every possible help to make this revision an interesting and not a laborious task.

1973                                                              M.E.

# Contents

# INTRODUCTION

"The most important biological function of Women is the reproduction of the race'. This introductory sentence to the first edition of 'A Way to Natural Childbirth' written by Mrs Heardman in April 1948 has been valid from the beginning of time and is still valid today. Civilisation and cultural developments have, however, changed a woman's position in society. Educational developments have contributed to the fact that women have an important part to play in the public and cultural life of the human race so that 'reproduction of the race' is no longer the sole contents and purpose of a woman's life. It is therefore sad to think that so many young women embark upon their first pregnancy unaware of the physiological and psychological changes that are involved. Preparation at school and at home during adolescence in many cases is still quite inadequate. Many are not even fully aware of the physiological events that may lead to pregnancy and the education for the responsibility involved in creating a new life is very often sadly neglected. Unfortunately the pleasures of sexual relationship are often over emphasized during these instruction periods. Self-expression which includes sexual expression is stressed and information is concentrated on the various methods of avoiding pregnancy. It very often fails to stress that full human self-expression if it leads to sexual relationship is only justified if it is the expression of a loving relationship. It must accept the partner as a real friend and not only as a member of the opposite sex. If this mutual respect for a human relationship is absent, sexual relationship is degraded to sexual promiscuity and is bound to lead to physical and emotional problems. It is something that 'happens' and not something that is planned and entered upon consciously. A young married woman may have dreamt of having a baby but when she realises that she really has conceived, this realisation comes to many as a surprise and very often as an unexpected one.

It is therefore important to give all available help during these early days to the young woman to accept pregnancy with all its physiological as well as emotional changes. She must be helped towards an attitude of active cooperation in which she retains a certain amount of voluntary decision. These problems will not only involve herself but also the relationship with her husband, social as well as financial adaptations may be necessary. The development of medical Science during the past decades has contributed enormously to the safety of mother and child, social legislation offers a great deal of help to the expectant mother, the modern concept of education for childbirth hopes to contribute to the solution of some of the physical and emotional problems of the events of the childbearing cycle. The three phases of this cycle are Pregnancy, Labour and the post-natal period or Puerperium. They must be seen in perspective and their true relationship must be emphasized. Labour must not be singled out as the most important event. Balanced perception of all events of the whole cycle will help the young woman to grow to greater physical as well as emotional maturity.

## Definition of Natural Childbirth

Childbirth is a natural physiological function. It may be sometimes more sometimes less comfortable, but if carried out by a healthy, normal person should be associated with satisfaction and a sense of achievement. Education for natural childbirth should create greater awareness of the interaction of mind and body, it should help the young mother to gain confidence that she will be able to cooperate with all members of the Obstetric Team. This demands a certain amount of knowledge of the events of pregnancy, labour and the puerperium. It will demand a certain amount of practice to lead to physical awareness. It will not result in perfect muscles or perfect breathing or perfect relaxation as isolated skills. It should enable every woman to go through pregnancy, labour and the puerperium in a state of mind in which she had complete command of herself and any avoidable emotional and physical damage has been prevented.

It is hoped that the contents of this little book will represent a modest contribution to help the young mother to live consciously through all the events of the childbearing cycle.

## Chapter 2

### Health Education during Childhood and Adolescence

Though much of what will be said in this chapter and throughout the book will refer more especially to women, it is likely that in future men will become, and rightly, much more interested in this subject.

Health education will be discussed, therefore, for both sexes and will be grouped under two main headings although both are interrelated. Physical education is the education of the child's body and mental education is the education of the child's mind, consisting of general biological education and specific sex education.

### Physical education

Dr Kathleen Vaughan in her book, *Safe Childbirth* states that there are three fundamental physical requirements for natural childbirth:

(1) Round (pelvic) brim (bones).
(2) Flexible joints (bones and joints).
(3) Natural postures (bones, joints, muscles).

The bones, joints, muscles and nervous pathways of the human body develop with the activities in which the child is engaged.

For the pre-school child it will be necessary in the future to make arrangements for both boys and girls to give ample opportunity for the normal pursuits of childhood, i.e. opportunities to climb and get over obstacles, open spaces free from the danger of traffic for free running, jumping and throwing. Indoor spaces where squatting for long periods is possible during pursuits to develop mental faculties. These play facilities both indoor and outdoor are essential to provide adequate growth stimuli for mental and physical development. The fact must be accepted that in future many young couples will live in flats in built up areas where natural open spaces are absent. Scientific research has provided ample proof that 'play' is an essential factor in the full development of the young of all species, both human and animal. Local Authorities as well as young parents must become aware of these basic necessities if serious damage to the development both mental and physical of future generations is to be avoided.

During school life these same 'play' facilities must be present both for mental as well as physical development. When a child sits for long periods indoors over lessons its general physical development will seriously suffer. Running, jumping, climbing and throwing are basic activities essential for the full physical development. This is particularly important for girls as the muscles essential to carry out these activities influence the development and shape of the female pelvis.

## Mental education

*General biological education.* In the school of to-day adequate instruction in biology is provided from the earliest years and right through the school, though the co-operation of the parents is vital too. Many excellent books exist for the parents to use for the school and pre-school child. (Three examples are cited in the Bibliography, Nos. 7, 11, 22.) When properly presented, young and old find the study of the biological functions of the human body a source of interest and wonder.

A certain prudery still exists in some people about bodily functions, and this may lead to inhibitions in adult life, affecting marriage and pregnancy; it also tends to prevent these people, if they become parents, from helping their children to acquire satisfactory knowledge in this subject.

*Specific sex education.* Again, it is not the purpose of this manual to enter into detail regarding this part of the subject which is dealt with in many admirable textbooks (Bibliography, Nos. 2, 14). Suffice it to say that children of all ages take a real interest in their normal bodily functions, asking questions at very early ages which are often a source of embarrassment to a less frank generation. As an example, B. asked at the age of 2½ years, 'Where did I come from?' and at

5 years, 'How did I get out?' and at 7 years, 'How did I get in?' She must have instructed her sister T., who said suddenly, at 4½ years, when told of the advent of another baby, that she wished she 'could peep into your tummy and see what he looks like.'

The principle in dealing with any anatomical or physiological question from a child is to be truthful (within the child's understanding) and matter of fact, and never to offer information beyond what has been asked. If children can grow up with animals and see as a matter of course baby chicks, kittens, puppies, calves, lambs, etc., around them, or, better still, be members of an enlarging family with new babies to look forward to and welcome, and to watch feeding naturally at the breast, having at the same time the information for which they seek with such lively interest imparted to them, there will be little difficulty in instructing them in adolescence. Such children find no difficulty either in later life during courtship, marriage, and pregnancy in maintaining the natural attitude with their parents which their early training engendered. If parents really cannot achieve the necessary candid un-embarrassed attitude to questions, they will no doubt in these days be answered at school, but this is very definitely second best.

No girl or boy should be allowed to approach the changes of adolescence without timely warning, and each sex should learn about the other. The boy and girl should learn at the appropriate time how to conduct themselves in mixed friendships. They should learn also that there is a mental and spiritual, as well as a physical, aspect of courting and mating, and that there is a great art in living together. They thus approach marriage and parenthood equipped to make them a success, and so create the home and the family which is the birthright of every child.

# Chapter 3

## Preparation during Pregnancy

It is still not a universal state of affairs to find the pregnant woman really well instructed in her bodily functions, and still less so in phenomena of pregnancy, labour, lactation and the puerperium. She has still far too often gained what little knowledge she has from hearsay, novels, plays, the cinema and television. Consciously or subconsciously she is still often afraid that she is facing an ordeal by pain which may even endanger her life. The fact that she is to experience a physiological muscular effort which can be as satisfying as playing a hard set of tennis or completing her washing and spring cleaning would cause her intense surprise. When it is put to her that a man who is to row in a boat race enters a period of very strict training beforehand, toils through the race with anything but apparent enjoyment, collapses over the oars at the end, and does it for the *sense of achievement* it gives him, she may begin to see light. If a man so trains for the combined mental and muscular effort, how can it be explained that we still allow women whose function it is to produce a new human life by mental and muscular effort, to embark upon this task often without any real training—and in *fear?* The analogy may be pressed still further: the man who rows the race is followed by his coach, who exhorts him to further efforts and corrects his faults etc. as the race proceeds. So the woman should have beside her during labour, and always available, a friendly, sympathetic and well informed professional councellor.

Women who are invited to attend training classes during pregnancy with the promise of such help, attend so readily and with such enjoyment that it becomes evident that this is the right course to pursue. This section will therefore deal at some length with the conduct of such classes and the instruction which should be given as a minimum.

No woman should be accepted to attend the classes without the consent of her medical adviser, and it is assumed that every woman will be receiving adequate antenatal supervision throughout pregnancy from a doctor either privately or at a clinic or in hospital.

The classes can begin when the doctor advises—it has however been proved useful to hold one early class in about the thirteenth to sixteenth week to deal with early problems such as diet, posture, breathing and planning for the future. The further training can then be continued after approximately six months, which is commonly the time when working women discontinue regular occupation.

The classes should be large enough for companionship to be adequate, and small enough for an atmosphere to develop in which any question or observation which a member wishes to make can be uttered. A dozen should, if possible be the maximum and half a dozen usually the minimum, though either fewer or more can prove satisfactory in the right hands.

A blanket or rug, a pillow and a chair (or stool) for each woman are all that is needed and a clean floor. A lavatory must be within easy reach and the women should be instructed to use it before the class. No special dress is needed, but suspender belts and girdles must be removed as well as shoes.

It is most satisfactory if every member of a class is about the same number of weeks pregnant. Sometimes this is however not possible, particularly in country districts. Under such conditions, a special effort should be made to teach breathing exercises and posture individually but otherwise let the women join whenever it is possible. No woman should join a class for the first time during instruction for labour.

## FIRST CLASS

This is the class which should be arranged early in pregnancy to deal with diet, posture, breathing and planning for the future.

### Diet

More detailed information may be given either by the doctor or the health visitor or the midwife. Adequate diet throughout pregnancy is very important, particularly as overeating must be avoided. There is often a tendency to gain too much weight, which is not beneficial and makes it more difficult to regain the figure and normal weight after the baby is born. The diet should contain plenty of protein i.e. meat, fish, cheese, eggs and milk and adequate amounts of fresh fruit and vegetables including salads. Starchy foods such as bread, potatoes, cakes and starchy sweets should only be eaten in moderation as these are primarily responsible for the excessive weight gain.

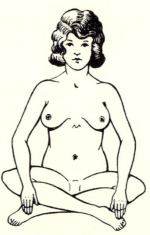

Figure 1

The register should be taken at the beginning of the class to keep an account of the number of attendances of each individual mother. This time should be spent by the mothers sitting on the floor in cross leg sitting with the hands lightly resting on the knees.

The time is used to relax the adductors of the hip joint so that the mother eventually can let the knees rest comfortably on the floor.

They are told that *labour* literally means *hard work* but also that it means controlled work. In order to be able to cope with it, they must become perfect in the preparatory work and this implies practice at home of the exercises learnt in classes. Every effort must be made to help the mothers to fit the exercises into their daily working routine and, by performing daily tasks correctly, to use them as exercises. It is explained that the baby is in a pearshaped muscular bag (uterus) and that the narrow end of the pear (the neck of the uterus) is facing downwards towards the birth canal. Labour takes place in three stages—the first stage serves to open up the neck and birth canal—the second stage involves the hardest work for the

**THE POSITION OF THE BABY IN THE MOTHER AT THE END OF PREGNANCY**

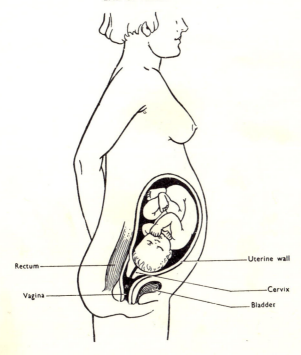

Rectum

Vagina

Uterine wall

Cervix

Bladder

Figure 2

mother when she must get to work to help to push the baby out—the third stage consists of the expulsion of the placenta or afterbirth which is the spongelike structure through which the baby has drawn its nourishment from the mother while contained in the uterus. Much more detail will be given later. This background is however necessary for the mother to appreciate the importance of diet and of breathing exercises as the air taken in through the lungs serves to burn up and make available the food eaten by the mother.

It must also be explained that correct posture during pregnancy is very important to avoid damage for the future to the back and backache during pregnancy.

Fig. 2 shows the position of the baby in relation to the mother.

Fig. 3 shows the position of the uterus in the pelvis. The pelvis is the keystone to human posture and the muscles which

**THE PELVIS SHOWING THE UTERUS**

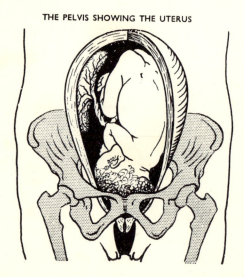

Figure 3

control its position are very important, these are the buttock muscles at the back and the abdominal muscles in the front.

## Exercise 1. Pelvic Tilting

### Lie on the back with knees bent

(1) Tighten the glutei and simultaneously draw in the lower abdominal wall, pressing the back firmly on to the floor. *N.B.* The part to draw in is that *directly above the pubic bones;* this requires care as most women will draw in the part under the ribs much more easily and this is useless for pelvic tilting. (Fig. 4a).

(2) Relax both groups of muscles and gently contract the lower back muscles to make a tunnel under them (Fig. 4b).

After attempting this several times find the anterior superior iliac spines, (the bones above either hip in front) and

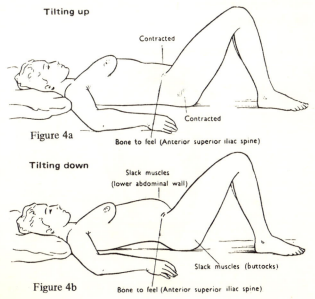

Tilting up

Contracted

Figure 4a

Contracted

Bone to feel (Anterior superior iliac spine)

Tilting down

Slack muscles
(lower abdominal wall)

Slack muscles (buttocks)

Figure 4b    Bone to feel (Anterior superior iliac spine)

test whether these go down towards the feet with the hollow back and come up towards the head with the flat one. If so the pelvis is tilting.Illustrate it with the articulated pelvis. Say that the movement is important in labour, as subsequent lessons will show, but is important immediately for good posture and correct carrying of the child (foetus).

## Alternative Position for 'Pelvic Tilting'

Once the above exercise had been learned, it may be more

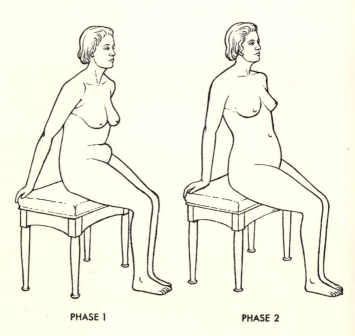

PHASE 1                    PHASE 2

Figure 5

convenient to practise it during the day in the following manner:

*Sitting forward on a stool with hands grasping the back of the stool.*

It is essential to sit forward on the stool to allow some of the weight to be taken on the feet. The position of the hands fixes the thoracic spine and therefore isolates the movement to the lumbar region.

Contract the gluteal and abdominal muscles to tilt the pelvis backwards; contract the back extensors and hip flexors to tilt the pelvis in the opposite direction—return to the starting position.

## EXERCISE 2 Breathing

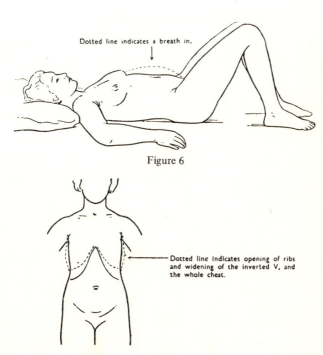

Dotted line indicates a breath in.

Figure 6

Dotted line indicates opening of ribs and widening of the inverted V, and the whole chest.

Figure 7

*Lie on the back with knees bent and feet on the floor, mouth closed.*

(1) Breathe gently in and out, keeping quite loose and letting

the abdominal wall rise up with the indrawn breath and drop down with the outgoing one. This must be practised *every day* until it can be done at any speed and to any depth, aiming at taking half a minute to draw in and then slowly breathe out (Fig.6).

(2) With mouth closed breathe in to expand the ribs sideways, opening out the inverted V of the ribs in front. Again, let the breath come out gently. Do this daily (Fig. 7)

## EXERCISE 3 Relaxation

Lie on the floor on one side, head only on the pillow, under arm behind the back and bent at the elbow, top arm lying on the floor or pillow in front. The top leg should be bent at hip, knee, and ankle, and placed in front of the bottom leg, which should be bent in the same manner (Fig. 8).

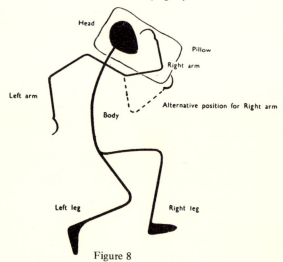

Figure 8

The three principles of relaxation are explained:

*1. Full support.* Gained in this case by the chosen position which deliberately places every limb and part of the body on a firm surface, so ensuring that no muscles have to *work* to hold any part in position. If difficulty is found with this position put further cushions under any uncomfortable parts, but practice on a firm surface.

*2. Lack of tension.* All joints being partially bent ensures that no muscle is unwittingly drawn taut across a joint. Eyes and mouth must be gently closed, and face and throat muscles consciously sagged.

*3. Mental peace.* To displace disturbing or worrying thoughts some positive idea must be given to the mind. Rhythm is a mental release, and the natural breathing rhythm serves the purpose. The mother is told to follow her own breathing by some symbol in her mind such as 'in-out' or 'up-down,' etc., and to use every effort to keep this up, thus literally listening to her own breathing. The same symbol should be used all the time.

As most individuals have little idea whether their muscles are relaxed or not, it is well to work up the body systematically, contracting each group of muscles in turn and releasing them until the whole body understands. This can be done as follows (the reader is referred to *Progressive Relaxation,* see Bibliography, No. 9, upon which the suggestions are based).

**Left leg**
    Squeeze down the toes—relax.
    Bend down the ankle—relax.
    Bend up the ankle—relax.
    Straighten the knee a little way—relax.
    Bend the knee a little way—relax.
    Tighten the hip muscle that you sit on—relax.
**Right leg**
    Do the same with the right leg in turn.
**Left arm**
    Stretch the fingers—relax.
    Bend elbow a little way—relax.
    Straighten elbow a little way—relax.
    Tighten the shoulder muscle on which you are lying—relax.
**Right arm**
    Do the same.

Then, after sagging the face and body as a whole, change from the natural breathing and begin to use the breathing (1) of exercise 2 as slowly and carefully as possible. If relaxation is good, a feeling as of the floor rising under the body like a lift will be experienced and a sensation of being weightless. If the time is suitable sleep will follow, and in any case there will be a delightful sensation of ease and comfort. The best time to practise is at night and daily after lunch during the afternoon rest.

All instructions should be given quietly and slowly and so that the voice is gradually lowered. When the end is reached, it should be explained very simply that this state of controlled relaxation is nature's desire for the first stage of labour and must be used each time the uterus contracts. Only thus can the long uterine muscle fibres act to open the cervix freely. The mother therefore has it in her own hands to aid her baby's door to open. A woman is extremely suggestible during relaxation, and only positive and helpful instruction must be given when relaxed.

Next, explain that during relaxation the circulation is at its slowest and the heart must be brought back carefully to its work, so small muscle movements, like clenching hands and feet, must be done, followed by stretching of limbs and a gradual sitting up, before standing once more.

## Relaxation of parts (iocalised) as a preparation

Some women will require further help with relaxation, and can generally appreciate it best after trying local relaxation of the main muscle groups; suggestions for these are now set out for the Teacher.

## Localised relaxation.

Using the lying position already described, concentrating on one joint at a time.

### Foot

Hold the leg above the ankle with one hand and ask the mother to dorsiflex the ankle while giving resistance over the dorsum with the other hand. Touch the dorsiflexors so that the mother knows which muscles are being used, then ask her to stop working and appreciate relaxation. Try plantar flexion in the same way. When the idea is fully understood ask her to 'relax' the foot, then test her ability by moving it up and down; it should be completely flabby.

### Knee

The same procedure can be adopted for flexion and extension of the knee.

### Hips

The same procedure will be effective here too. The other leg can be educated and tested.

### Head

Ask the mother to press the head back against a hand placed on the occiput to appreciate the work of the extensors of the head, then stop pressing. Repeat this with a hand on the forehead to appreciate the action of the flexors.

### Throat

While the head is pressed back let her try opening and closing the mouth to feel the tension and relaxation on the throat muscles.

### Face

Without any resistance try in turn various expressions of the face and then relaxation of them.

1. Lifting the eyebrows and making the forehead wrinkle horizontally.
2. Drawing the eyebrows together and frowning.
3. Screwing the eyes up very tight.
4. Wrinkling up the nose.
5. Showing the top teeth by drawing up the upper lip.
6. Showing the bottom teeth by drawing down the lower lip.
7. Pursing the lips.
8. Blowing out the cheeks with closed mouth.

Next it would be wise to apply the principles of relaxation

to lying on the back (described later in Exercise 13), and in this position to attempt local relaxation of the arms.

## Hand

Ask the mother to make a fist, then hold round the forearm with one hand and place the other over the fingers. Ask her to open the fingers against the pressure. Repeat with the wrist.

## Elbow

Get the elbow bent at right angles, and hold the upper arm. Ask the mother first to bend the elbow against resistance; point out the elbow flexors and then get her to relax them. Repeat the same procedure with the elbow extensors.

## Shoulder

Get the mother to lift the arm at the shoulder still further sideways along the pillows and against some resistance and then cease the work. Repeat the procedure, resisting the return. She will thus appreciate the work of the abductors and adductors.

## Hips

Get the mother to press her bent knees firmly together against resistance of both hands, one on the inside of each knee simultaneously. Point out that when she relaxes the knees will fall apart. Resist now on the outer side of both knees, getting the knees still wider, then letting them return to the natural width apart.

## Head

Put a hand on on one side of the head and get the mother first to press sideways against it, and when the relaxation from that is appreciated, get her to try turning the head and relaxing it on both sides.

It will be obvious that this will be too big an undertaking in one class. Indeed, from experience few pregnant women seem to need much help once the general principles are grasped. Those that do need it are best kept back for a few minutes after a class, and the way the resistance is given should be explained to them so that they can get a similar type of help at home.

Throughout this localised contraction and relaxation it should be pointed out that breathing should be natural and easy, and it helps if it is kept as a conscious and very rhythmic affair.

## EXERCISE 4. Posture Correction
### (Started by Pelvic Tilting)

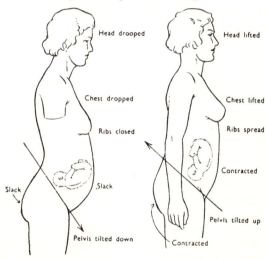

The tilted down pelvis with baby using the abdominal muscles as a hammock and causing them to be stretched. The weight falls on the back muscles which become strained and lead to the well-known backache of pregnancy.

The abdominal muscles holding the baby in the tilted-up pelvis. A perfect balance of muscle back and front.

Figure 9                    Figure 10

Get the mothers to stand and try out pelvic tilting on the lines of the accompanying sketches (Figs. 9, 10).
Pelvic tilting is particularly valuable for the prevention of

*backache* during pregnancy, which is both one of the commonest and one of the most tiresome accompaniments. Experience has shown that backache is extremely rare in mothers attending training classes.

When the pelvic tilting is appreciated use the rib-spread breathing (Exercise 2. Breathing (2) to open out the chest, and finally experiment with a lift of the head towards the roof, as if a piece of string were tied to the very top of the head and fixed to the ceiling. Point out the necessity for a firm stance with *all* toes pressed against the floor and weight well over the arches. A woman carrying a child should be noticeable for her good looks, health, happiness, and poise of body.

*N.B.* If this is found to be difficult practise posture correction first, lying on the floor until proficient (p. 59) then try it sitting and finally standing.

## Planning for the Future

Prenatal instruction in the preparation for the 'Motherhood role' has a very important part to play to help expectant mothers to manage their new responsibilities more successfully and thus reduce the post-partum emotional stress. This preparation should however not only be confined to physical and intellectual preparation, the mother must also be given the opportunity to think ahead and plan for changes which will arise.

One of the most important factors is to prepare financially for a period when the income of the family may be reduced due to the fact that the wife who previously contributed to the family income cannot do so for a considerable time after the baby is born. It is important to discuss with the expectant mother the fact of laying a foundation for the baby's security in future life by attending to the baby's needs *herself* for a considerable time unless satisfactory and continuous arrangements can be made with a relation such as mother or mother in law. Not facing up to these problems may contribute to develop a feeling of guilt in the mother which again is detrimental to her emotional stability. Where necessary she should be helped to budget her future expenses and also be advised of any financial help that is available to her. It will also be reassuring to her to be informed that part of her emotional instability is due to endocrine imbalance and will right itself during the next few months and therefore constitutes a passing phase. Suddenly bursting into tears when one has not done so before is upsetting for both marriage partners and it is reassuring to know why one suddenly has lost one's mental balance. So much theoretical information is now available in book and pamphlet form that it is confusing to many young mothers. What once may have been an instinctive attitude has often been lost in civilized society and often needs a guiding hand to sort it out. The responsibilities of motherhood can be learned.

Another problem to be faced is that man is a social animal and needs social contacts. We need to have an outlet for our doubts and queries, discuss them with others in a similar position. This is one of the benefits of antenatal classes. The expectant mother learns to appreciate that she is not a unique phenomenon. The husband is of course one of the most important contacts but it is also very beneficial to make friends of other couples who are in a similar position. In-laws can be of great help if they are made to realize that they are friends to the young people and not an authority. To maintain outside interests is of tremendous importance. Early arrangements for a baby-sitter perhaps once a week prevents a feeling of isolation and the baby becoming a burden instead of a joy. Mothers, Mothers-in-law, friends—all can help, but it needs planning beforehand.

Perhaps considering these problems, bringing them up to conscious level may help to lay the foundation to happier and lasting family relationships and also to happier and less dissatisfied young people.

## SECOND CLASS

### (24th/28th week of pregnancy)

The previously taught four exercises of the early class are revised and faults which may have crept in are corrected.

## EXERCISE 5. Contraction and Relaxation of Pelvic Floor Muscles

*Lie on the back with knees bent and feet flat on the floor.*
(Later this can be done, allowing the knees to part gently during relaxation, but feet are kept together).

Take this in three stages:

(1) Squeeze the two buttock muscles (glutei) together, counting one to six slowly. Relax to the same number of counts. Do this until the action is strong and perfect.

(2) While doing (1) press the thighs firmly together at the back, and pull up as though preventing a bladder action, and lengthen the counts to seven for both actions together. Repeat until perfect.

(3) While doing (1) and (2) draw in the back passage (anus) very strongly as if to prevent a bowel action. Lengthen the counts to ten for all three actions together.

Point out that the pelvic floor muscles *must* be elastic for natural childbirth, so that the child may pass through comfortably and painlessly. Muscle is *living elastic* and unlike the commercial variety, becomes more elastic with careful and repeated contraction and relaxation. This exercise therefore prepares the way, but is never actually used in labour. It should, however, be done daily, and can be practised quite easily standing with heels and *toes together* whilst washing up, cooking, waiting in queues, etc., also in sitting.

## EXERCISE 6. Side Bending in the Spine

(By Moving a Leg and Tilting the Pelvis Sideways)

The skin and muscles of the abdomen gradually stretch during pregnancy, so does a fibrous band, called the linea alba, lying between the muscles which run vertically on either side of the centre line. This class will deal with these facts.

*Muscles of the abdomen.* These run in three directions on each side, as shown in Figure 11. Their different slants allow them to move the trunk in different directions, i.e. to bend forward, bend sideways, or to turn. It has already been seen that the baby is held in place by all of them working together,

therefore they must remain strong and elastic during pregnancy. Exercise 1 has used the muscles straight. Exercise 6 will
use the muscles to bend the trunk sideways, and Exercise 7
will use them to turn the trunk (Figs. 12 and 13).

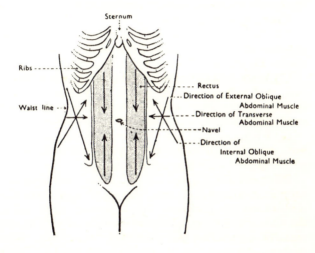

Figure 11

*Lie on the back with one knee bent and one straight.* Draw up
the straight leg along the ground, making the waist line firm
and much more curved inwards, push the leg back along the
floor in the reverse direction. Do this with the other leg also
(Fig. 12).

## EXERCISE 7 Turning in the Spine

### (By Moving a Leg and Rotating the Pelvis)

Use the same position to start, but roll the bent knee *over*
the straight to try and get the knee on to the floor, i.e. if the
right knee is used it must get to the floor on the left side of
the left leg. This must be done by the muscles of the waist line

and not by those of the groins (adductors) by mistake. Finish by allowing the knee to relax gently outward to the floor on its own side (Fig. 13).

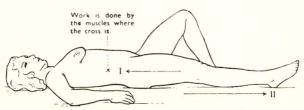

Work is done by the muscles where the cross is.

x   1

II

The straight leg is drawn along the floor in the direction of arrow I. and then pushed down in the direction of arrow II.   The movement in the spine can be increased by moving the head and shoulders towards the right leg, reaching down it with the right arm.

Figure 12

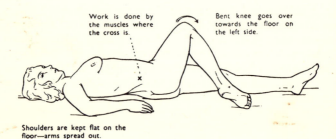

Work is done by the muscles where the cross is.

Bent knee goes over towards the floor on the left side.

x

Shoulders are kept flat on the floor—arms spread out.

Figure 13

## Care of the Skin

Using some oil on the hands as a lubricant (olive, odourless castor, or liquid paraffin will do), *(a)* rub the hands firmly all over the abdomen (five minutes), *(b)* pick up as much of the skin covering the abdomen as possible and pass it from one hand to the other to lift if off the underlying muscle (five minutes). This may help to render the skin more elastic and is valuable in reducing the irritation which is sometime felt in the last few weeks as a result of the stretching of the skin.

## Stretching of the Linea Alba

This cannot be prevented and stretches to an average of 4 inches. Not being elastic it cannot return to its former state as the muscles can, and so it can be the cause of a protruding abdomen after childbirth if the mother does not know how to keep her abdominal muscles in good condition and to tone up her rectus muscles so that they can meet and obliterate the gap. This will be dealt with in Chapter 6.

All the usual exercises should be practised as well as the new ones.

## THIRD CLASS

### (29th Week of Pregnancy)

Breathing exercises should be included in every class and posture checked at the end of each session.

## EXERCISE 8. Squatting

Flace the feet down flat on the floor and about 18 inches apart parallel, holding on to a firm support (e.g. the sink). Squat right down on to the heels, starting with outward rotation of the knees. The balance may be difficult to acquire, but every day it will be easier, and some small job like cleaning the shoes, peeling potatoes, tidying a drawer should be done in squatting. If it is difficult to begin with, wear shoes with flat heels at first.

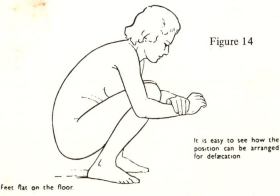

Figure 14

It is easy to see how the position can be arranged for defæcation

Feet flat on the floor

This is the position which primitive women naturally assume during labour because it is the one in which it is easiest to push the baby out of the pelvis. Getting accustomed to this position during pregnancy, by regular and repeated squatting, makes it easier for the mother to do her work during the second stage of labour in the modified position which is now used, because the mother is more comfortable lying in bed tipped back against two or more pillows then she would be balancing on her feet on the ground, and the muscle and joint action is the same. During pregnancy it may also help to relieve constipation. The use of foot-stools or boxes in front of the lavatory seat may be useful to put the muscle of expulsion in the position of maximum effort.

## EXERCISE 9. Pelvic Tilting

### (Variations of Exercise 1)

*1. On the hands and knees.* The hands below the shoulders and the knees below the hips, keeping all angles true right angles (Fig. 15).

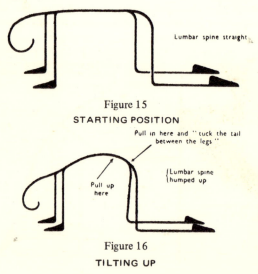

Lumbar spine straight

Figure 15

STARTING POSITION

Pull in here and " tuck the tail between the legs "

Pull up here

Lumbar spine humped up

Figure 16

TILTING UP

The pelvis is tilted by alternately tightening the glutei (hip muscles) and the lower abdominal wall and then relaxing them, the body assuming first a humped-up appearance and then the back straightening again (Figs. 15 and 16)

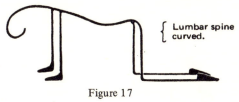

{ Lumbar spine curved.

Figure 17

**INCORRECT POSITION**

*Warning.* This exercise should not be carried to the point where the spine becomes hollowed (Fig. 17).

2. *Kneeling.* The forearms crossed on the seat of a chair, knees well under the chair, hips on heels. (Fig. 18).

3. *Sitting.* Knees and feet wide apart with forearms crossed and resting on pillows on a table. The pelvis is then tilted by contracting the hip and abdominal muscles alternately with releasing them (Fig. 19).

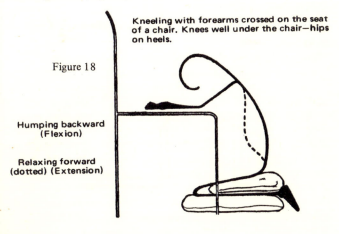

Figure 18

Humping backward (Flexion)

Relaxing forward (dotted) (Extension)

Kneeling with forearms crossed on the seat of a chair. Knees well under the chair—hips on heels.

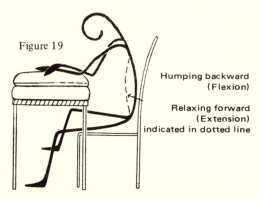

Figure 19

Humping backward
(Flexion)

Relaxing forward
(Extension)
indicated in dotted line

The exercises have value for strengthening the abdominal muscles and for improving the posture. They will also be of indirect value in the second stage, and may be of value in the first stages of labour as an alternative to relaxation or in combination with it. Variation (2) may be of value as an alternative position for 'bearing down' in the second stage. These alternatives will be explained in the Eigth Class (p. 43).

## FOURTH CLASS
### (30th Week of Pregnancy)

**EXERCISE 10. Polishing the Floor on Hands and Knees**
**On hands and knees**
Move around the room dusting or polishing the floor.

The abdominal organs are all attached to the backbone by strong membranes. In this position these organs hang from the backbone like clothes on a line, instead of hanging, as they do when you are upright, like a flag on a pole. When they are like a flag on a pole they tend to fall down towards the pelvis and press on the great blood vessels and nerves. This hands and knees position relieves that pressure. Moving around in this position strengthens the abdominal muscles which is desirable in pregnancy. Taking up this position in labour very often relieves the painful pressure on the blood vessels and nerves caused by the contracting uterus when lying on the back.

## EXERCISE 11. Breathing (3)

Breathing exercises are gradually developed throughout the classes and the exercise described here is a further development of Exercise 2.

*Lie on the back with knees bent and feet on the floor, mouth slightly open.*

(3) Breath in more quickly, lifting up the sternum, or breast bone, letting it lower again. *Normal* every day breathing should of course, be done through the nose with the mouth closed. This type of breathing should however now be practised as an exercise as it is used during the later part of labour. It is shallower and therefore quicker and breathing through the nose is comparatively slower.

All three breathing exercises can be done in the bath, or in bed before getting up or going to sleep at night, or during the midday rest. They are important because the mother's most important work during labour is accomplished by her controlled breathing.

If practised apart from other exercises each type of breathing *must not be done more than three times.*

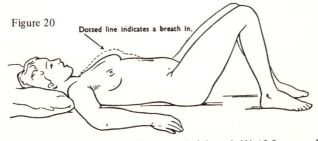

Figure 20

Dotted line indicates a breath in.

The previously taught Exercise 2 (1) and (2) if frequently practised will help the mother to avoid become uncomfortably breathless during slight exertion.

## Muscle control

Some conscious control of isolated muscle groups will already have been introduced at the beginning of the course when teaching general relaxation. More difficult coordination and conscious attempt of contracting and releasing tension in various muscle groups can now be attempted in order to prepare for the final cooperation and control during labour. The mother must be able during the final expulsive effort to contract the abdominal muscles with complete simultaneous relaxation of the adductor muscles of the thigh and of the pelvic floor.

The mother has previously learned to contract elbow flexors and knee flexors, the following progression is suggested:

*Lying.* Contracting of elbow and knee flexors of one side of the body followed by release.

This exercise should be repeated by giving quick unexpected commands to either side of the body.

*Lying.* Contraction of the muscles of one upper and one lower limb on opposite sides of the body—followed by complete release, e.g. left arm with right leg.

**Final practice.** *Lying with knees bent, feet resting on the floor:* parting of the knees into complete abduction by releasing the tone in the adductors of the thigh and the pelvic floor muscles with simultaneous contraction of the abdominal muscles.

The mother can learn to realise the lack of contraction in the adductor muscles by placing one hand on the inside of the thigh and the other hand on the abdomen in order to feel the contraction of the abdominal muscles.

### Supervision of progress

All previous exercises are checked carefully before introducing any new ones. Mothers will usually have been found to have done so well by home practice that *two to three* new ideas can be introduced.

### Social period

It is ideal if a cup of tea or any hot drink can now be provided and free discussion take place. The instructor can either speak privately to answer queries or skilfully use a question to draw the whole group into the picture. This should be the procedure at each class. It will not therefore be mentioned again.

### FIFTH CLASS
(31st Week of Pregnancy)

## EXERCISE 12. Breathing Variations

It will be found during labour that the mother's part, in physical terms, consists almost wholly of a control of breathing. After running through the breathing exercises described in Exercises 2 and 11, take the following variations:

### 4. Lying on the back with the knees bent

Open the mouth and draw a deep quick breath, using methods (1) and (2) described on page 15, then close the mouth and hold the breath, counting ten slowly. At the end of this period let the breath go naturally and rapidly (it will make a noise like a deep sigh). Immediately repeat two or three times. Practise holding the breath for longer and longer periods.

5. In the same position and with mouth open draw a number of breaths as in method (3), first quick and shallow, second quick and deep; this creates a panting effect, the quick ones similar to a dog lying apparently breathless on a hot summer day, the deep ones similar to the breathing of an athlete who has run 100 yards to beat a record. It should make the abdomen vibrate up and down.

With concentration on breathing control the following information is given: As previously mentioned, labour is said to take place in three stages—first, second and third; throughout all three stages contractions of the uterus or womb (the muscle bag in which the baby lies) occur at regular intervals. These contractions are often still misnamed 'labour pains'. The uterus is not the only hollow organ in the body which expels its contents; both the rectum and the bladder do this in a comparable manner. Neither of these expulsive acts is normally accompanied by pain; rather they may be regarded as one of the primitive pleasures, as observation of any normal small child will prove. One of the reasons why this contraction of the uterus frequently may be painful is because, through ignorance women are afraid. The sensation of the uterine contraction will often be interpreted as pain, because the mother was told to expect pain. Emotions such as fear are frequently associated with the tightening of certain muscle fibres in hollow muscular organs. The uterus is no exception and the fibres affected are the fibres of the lower end of the uterus (the neck). These fibres should relax to allow widening of the neck. The contraction of the upper fibres of the uterus has now to overcome the resistance of the lower fibres and so the contractions push the baby against a resistance, and that hurts. This pain is intensified by fear. However, if a woman learns about her labour and realises that when the contractions occur, in a peaceful and happy atmosphere, she will find that in most cases she does not experience any sensation she is not prepared to meet.

The first stage of labour lasts until the neck is wide open, and then the mother must get to work and start pushing her baby out. This pushing further opens out the birth canal (vagina and vulva) and stretches the skin and muscles between the vulva and the anus (perineum). When she has done all this the second stage is at an end and the baby is born. The third stage consists of the coming of the placenta or afterbirth (which is the spongelike object through which the baby has drawn its food from the mother's womb), the bag of waters (this is also called the membranes and is the bag in which the baby has lived within the womb) and the cord (which has been attached to the placenta at one end and to the baby's navel at the other end and through which the nourishment passed).

## SIXTH CLASS
### (32nd Week of Pregnancy)

The essential physical basis having now been taught, the next step is to fit what has been learnt subjectively into the stages of labour objectively.

First, alternative positions for relaxation are practised, bearing in mind the three principles outlined in the first class.

### EXERCISE 13. Alternative Positions
for Relaxation

Lying on the back with a pillow under the head, two

pillows under the knees, a pillow supporting the feet. The arms should be bent at the elbows and at a little distance from the body each resting on a pillow, and the head pillow should be raised up at each side of the head to prevent the head from rolling to either side (Fig. 21).

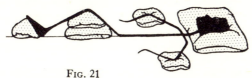

Fig. 21

In an armchair with feet on the floor or a footstool. Thighs fully supported, a pillow for the head, forearms supported along the arms of the chair (Fig. 22).

*Stage 1.*

The relaxation position in which the mother feels most comfortable is chosen, and each time a contraction of the uterus occurs (so-called 'labour pains') use the breathing method (1), Exercise 2. The contractions last on an average 30 seconds and are felt as a tensing of the abdomen and an *ache in the back*. The indrawn breath should move the abdominal wall outwards and should as nearly as possible last half of the time the uterus is contracting, the outgoing breath occupying the other half.

*With effective relaxation these do not become anything the mother is not prepared to experience.* They increase in strength, and the intervals between them decrease until the cervix is fully open (dilated).

During the later part of Stage 1 the mother will find that breathing using the abdominal wall during a contraction becomes almost impossible and is exhausting. She should now adopt a different procedure. During contraction: with rising contraction take a deep breath and immediately release air without abdominal effort. During continuing contraction upper chest breathing (Exercise 11 Breathing 3) should be carried out to the height of the contraction. When the contraction subsides revert to deeper abdominal breathing, when the contraction has completely passed away, make a

conscious expiratory effort (not forced) and then continue to breathe fully and quietly.
*Stage 2.*

After the cervix is dilated the baby is gradually expelled by the uterus. An active effort on the part of the mother may be called for to assist this action. She will probably lie on her back, her head and shoulders raised on pillows, and her knees bent exactly to the same degree as in the squatting (Exercise 8, page 25) but she may put her arm round her thighs or her knees.

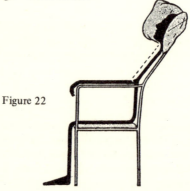

Figure 22

The effort is similar to the action of emptying the bowels but should be directed towards the vagina. The abdominal wall hardens and protrudes if the effort is correctly made. This 'pushing' can only be used as long as the contraction lasts, and then the mother must relax on her back, probably with the legs straight and spread apart, arms as in Relaxation (on the back). This is all repeated with each contraction until the baby is born. Point out that, quite unconsciously, pelvic tilting occurs alternately up when the knees are bent up, and down when the legs are straightened throughout Stage 2.

It will be noticed that the modified form of breathing used in the 'bearing down' action has not as yet been practised. There is, however, a natural daily action which takes place in a similar way—that is, the emptying of the bowels. If a stool of suitable height is placed in front of the lavatory seat and the feet put on this while the body is slightly stooped over and the head drooped (the squatting position of Exercise 8.), and the bowels are emptied by taking a breath and holding it and then bearing down, a daily practice of this second stage of labour becomes possible without strain. (*N.B.* In some cases it might be wise to give this information much earlier in pregnancy).

All the other Exercises 1 to 12 are checked.

Delivery procedures may vary and it is essential to ascertain the methods practised at the place of confinement, to ensure the full cooperation of the mother.

*Stage 3.*

The mother has no further part to play but to enjoy the fruits of her labour, and the more fully she is able to do this the more satisfactorily the afterbirth will come away.

The essential physical facts having now been fitted into labour, it is important to lay the mental (or emotional) foundations just as carefully.

The success of labour depends upon the mother grasping her reactions and feelings and realising that labour calls for control and skill and, like other physical feats, is a character-building undertaking.

*Stage 1.*

Just as a pregnant woman changes and tends to grow healthier, happier, and better looking, so during labour a woman changes and should know that this will be so. It is not uncommon that near the expected date, even for some weeks before, a feeling of impatience and frustration grows. Possibly it is nature's method of helping the desire for the child's birth. As labour starts this gives way to excitement and exhilaration, 'a wanting to tell everyone.' This lasts until about half dilation, the mother gradually becoming more serious and realising that her work has now inevitably to be done.

It is this inevitableness that at this stage brings some element of doubt and even fear into almost all women's minds.

What they have heard from friends and relations, what they have read, all tend to rise to the surface, and it is here-that the positive instruction of the classes serves them first. They know what they have to do, and because of their teaching and practice feel confident they can do it. They have appreciated uterine contractions probably for some weeks, and now realise that their accompaniment is a faint ache in the lower back, so slight that it may be ignored for hours and even throughout labour. If it grows in intensity it can be relieved by relaxation and firm pressure or rubbing, by the attendant, over the sacral region. Labour sensations are usually in the back, but may be in the front, and are what are known as 'referred sensations.' A well-prepared mother *with suitable attendance when she needs it* to exhort her to further effort and to encourage her or to correct her faults will contunue with her relaxation and gradually become aware herself of the onset of her second stage. She is taught that some or all of the following phenomena will be present.

## Transition stage (between stages 1 and 2)

1. *The contractions* will have narrowed down to round about *two or three minute intervals* and seem almost contin-uous. (The attendant will notice increasing amnesia between them.)

2. There will be a growing feeling of a *lump in the rectum* as of a very large motion to be passed. It is the pressure of the baby's head against the rectum. The sensation in the back gets lower and lower.

3. A *catch in the breath* comparable to a 'belch' appears at intervals. It is the first attempt of the diaphragm to establish an expulsive reflex.

4. It may produce a *nausea and desire* to vomit, and the mother should be warned to close her mouth and swallow, and bear downward very slightly to check the desire.

5. *Violent shaking* as if excited. Enough to make the teeth chatter in some cases and frighten the mother if not warned.

6. *Cramp* in the buttocks, thighs, or calves; stretching the legs between contrations will help.

7. *Inability to make the abdominal wall move by breathing* during a contraction, thus making abdominal breathing impossible.

*N.B.* The mother must *open her mouth* and change to the breathing of Exercise 12 (3) and continue to relax this way.

8. The mother finds herself *growing very hot.*

9. *Rupture of the membranes*, which may go with a distinct 'pop' but does not hurt.

*N.B.* The membranes can rupture before labour starts or at any time during labour as well.

10. *Increasing tenderness to touch* over the abdomen and back.

11. *A desire to empty the bowels* which, when irresistible, usually heralds the second stage. It is accompanied usually by *an involuntary bearing down movement of the abdominal wall*, never experienced at any other time, and most interesting and entertaining to feel if warned beforehand. It must not be used for bearing down until full dilation, and therefore the panting breathing of Exercise 12 (5) must be adopted to prevent the breath being held, or the abdomen held contracted.

*N.B.* The attendant may also notice:

12. The onset of, and increasing, *amnesia*, which often gives the *appearance* of exhaustion but this is not so.

13. An increase in, or the appearance of, a bloody *mucous discharge.* (The mother can feel this coming away.)

14. *The change in breathing* described under No. 7 can be clearly heard, and gradually the vocal cords tend to be used, producing an expulsive groan or grunt on expiration.

*Stage 2.*

Once her own suspicions are confirmed by the attendant and she is told that her cervix is fully open and she may begin to expel, she will experience a very great change. Whereas her whole being has been concentrating upon controlled relaxation, possibly in some trepidation, now she will find her personality changes and she becomes completely sure of herself and settles down to concentrate on a job which exists in a world of its own. This information will be most *effective* if given during the relaxation practice; it will have to be repeated several times in subsequent classes as it must be firmly imprinted.

Between bearing down efforts amnesia is often so marked that the mother will not hear questions or remarks, and she may profess herself 'too tired' to make any more effort as the stage goes on. All the same, each time a uterine contraction occurs the effort to bear down is resumed and the mother realises that she is growing heated and perspiring exactly as if she were playing a strenuous game. Gradually she begins to feel the child in the vagina instead of the rectum, and the time for which she has been waiting draws near. She knows that soon a very obvious stretching feeling will be experienced which sometimes amounts to a feeling of splitting open. This must not rouse alarm, as it is not painful when the muscles are well prepared; it should be *appreciated* as it is the prelude to the birth of the head. Round about this stage the mother may be turned on her side or left on her back, according to the wishes of the obstetrician, and she may be asked to pant softly as in Exercise 12, (5) instead of bearing down, so that the baby's head can be born more gently.

As the head is born she will feel her first sensation of release and can if she wishes watch the body come. Within minutes she may see the baby completely born, and here she has such a rush of feelings, physical and mental, joy and release and elation, that one cannot attempt to describe it to her. She will watch the baby's first movements, listen to its first cry, and as soon as the cord is cut she may hold it in her arms bundled up in its blanket, velvet soft and warm, in all its perfection.
*Stage 3.*

After a short period of waiting, during which full rein may be given to all thoughts and emotions, one further expulsive effort will produce the placenta and a third feeling of relief will be experienced. This is not really an anticlimax as some hold. it is a *physical* relief of quite surprising magnitude, and the delight in finding the abdomen flat once more has to be experienced to be believed. Here again the mother may be interested in seeing placenta and cord, and should ask to be shown it if she so desires.

When all this is over she will feel extremely fit and well and probably ravenously hungry and thirsty. She will respond to all suggestions happily and state herself ready to get up at once. She will want her baby near her, as soon as it is washed and dressed and comfortable, or even before.

This explanation is given whilst practising the physical counterparts of the stages, and the other exercises are again practised as usual.

## SEVENTH CLASS
(33rd Week of Pregnancy)

### Knowledge Versus Ignorance

At this point it is essential to make clear to the mother that nature seems to demand certain behaviour at certain periods of labour. A summary of the overall requirements of labour as far as the mother is concerned will prove more helpful than starting with details of the various stages of labour.

As labour in a primipara will usually last 12 to 15 hours, the most important factors are conservation of energy and a good oxygen supply for the working tissues.

*Early in the first stage.* Full relaxation and quiet abdominal breathing.

*Later in the first stage.* Full relaxation and abdominal and upper chest breathing.

Failure to follow this procedure may result in severe discomfort.

*In the transition between first and second stage.* Relaxation (in spite of the inability to move the abdomen extensively with breathing during contractions) must be maintained; breathing must pass into the chest, since moving the abdomen against nature's demand produces pain. Explanation has been given under Transition Stage earlier (p. 36) and if the mother knows that the period of time is now short before the onset of the second stage and the hard physical work, she will rest expectantly looking for the signs by which she can recognise its onset and therefore be in good condition to start expulsion at the right moment. This time is probably the most difficult part of labour, and it is here where back rubbing and or inhalation analgesia is of greatest benefit, if the mother has difficulty in continuing her relaxation. It must be impressed on the mother that she must never push unless told to do so.

*Early in the second stage.* Expulsion must be done at whatever strength the uterus urges, full relaxation of the pelvic floor muscles during abdominal contraction must have been practised during pregnancy. Failure to do this will lead to pain and may lead to inertia and inability to push at all.

*Later in the second stage.* (as the baby's head reaches the pelvic floor to stretch the vulva). Full relaxation of the pelvic floor and controlled breathing as directed. This is probably the second point of greatest difficulty in labour. Inability to conform with the instructions of the attendant at this point is one of the commonest reasons for the use of an anaesthetic which robs the mother of her consciousness and so of the supreme experience of the birth of her child.

*In the third stage.* Elation and happiness. If these are not present the mother is physically ill at ease. The uterus should contract firmly down upon the placenta. Being an involuntary muscle it can only be affected reflexly. The most effective method would appear to be the mother's mental state, acting reflexly through the autonomic nervous system (hence the value of natural childbirth and holding the child in her arms as soon as possible). This contraction of the uterine muscle expels the placenta.

*The start of labour* To continue with this class, the mother must now be instructed in the method of procedure when labour starts. First, it is important to emphasise that the *sensation,* if any, is a *backache* or *abdominal discomfort.* It is surprising how many women refuse to believe they are in labour because this is all they feel. It is difficult to give any hard and fast rule, so that it is well to suggest the main variations without any regard to the order in which they may occur.

1. A *show* A menstrual period appears to be starting, and there is a very slight show of blood-stained mucus often following a call to empty the bowels at a rather unusual time.

2. A *backache,* which comes and goes at regular intervals. This will certainly come sooner or later, and may follow the 'show' at once. It is accompanied by a hardening of the uterus which can be felt by putting the hands on the abdominal wall.

3. *Rupture* of the membranes with a gush of fluid or a continuous trickle. This occurs early in only a small percentage of women. If it occurs first, the mother should go to the hospital or nursing home at once, and if to be confined at home should send for the midwife or doctor who will give further instructions.

If (1) or (2) occur they may be noted, but the daily routine should continue. The important symptom is the contractions, and if they persist they should be timed. As soon as the interval is 10 minutes or less (and it may *start* at less) and lasts for approximately 15 to 20 seconds the mother should inform her doctor or midwife and go to hospital or nursing home according to where she is to be confined.

If the doctor has given the mother any instructions which conflict with the above for some reason she must, of course, follow his instructions implicitly.

In (1), (2), or (3) the class instructor may want to know so that she may meet the mother and make sure that she understands her procedure now that the event has begun, for just as an athlete in the excitement of the match can forget and make mistakes, so the mother can become confused. It is also understood in natural childbirth that no mother shall ever be left alone at any time when she wishes for company and expert help.

A taxi or ambulance should be ordered, giving approximate date, so that the name and address is familiar to the proprietor or authority.

The instructor tries to 'set the stage' for each mother according to her place of confinement and the method by which she will be delivered. This entails a knowledge on the part of the physiotherapist of the labour wards and the medical men's or midwives' methods. There are two important details concerning labour about which the mother should be warned.

(1) Rectal or vaginal examinations may be done—the former probably lying on her left side and the latter probably lying on her back; and they consist of the midwife or doctor inserting a gloved finger up the rectum or vagina to learn the amount of dilation which has occurred in the cervix.

(2) The foetal heart will be listened to with the stethoscope or ear, the mother lying flat on her back. The stethoscope may be of the small 'tin trumpet' variety or the well-known kind used by all doctors, or the examiner may lay an ear on the mother's abdomen.

When the onset of labour starts with a backache only, many women move about the house, garden and streets on their daily round and find that easy and natural. When however the contractions have settled down and occur at intervals of 7 to 10 minutes, have become quite strong and last from 20 seconds to one minute, the mother will no longer be able to ignore them. She will have to settle down to a routine during contractions. It is not essential to lie down unless this phase occurs during the night. The positions illustrated in Figure 21 or 22 may prove very comfortable. If the mother prefers to lie down the position shown in Figure 8 may be found comfortable. All these positions are tried out and the mother should breathe in quietly and deeply during rising contractions, concentrating on deep abdominal breathing (Exercise 1). At this stage some mothers prefer pelvic tilting during a contraction (generally kneeling on hands and knees, kneeling, sitting or even standing leaning on the table or mantelpiece). Many doctors and midwives are quite agreeable that the mother shall do whatever is most comfortable and suits her best.

## EIGHTH CLASS
### (34th Week of Pregnancy)

The contents of the last class is quickly revised and the rehearsal of labour continued as follows.

When the dilation is nearing the halfway stage, the contractions are much more forceful and last longer. At this stage the breathing rhythm during contractions must be changed in order to avoid pressure on the contracting uterus. With rising contraction the mother takes a deep breath and immediately releases the air without abdominal effort. During the continuing contraction she changes to upper chest breathing (Exercise 11, 3) to the height of the contraction, reverting at the end of the contraction to deeper breathing, breathing out without abdominal effort.

## Transition stage.

The mother will probably find herself now in the optimum delivery position for which she has been prepared by practising squatting correctly. (Exercise 8). She may now be asked to practice Breathing (Exercise 7, 5), or use Inhalation Analgesia to avoid pushing.

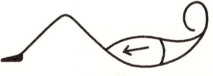

Figure 23

## Stage 2.

This is the phase for which the mother has conserved all her energy. At the beginning of a contraction, the mother must quickly check that her pelvic floor is fully relaxed and draw in a full breath through the open mouth, holding her breath, closing the mouth and curling the head forward. She now follows her attendants instruction 'to push' by contracting her abdominal muscles. Usually the uterine contraction lasts longer than the mother can hold her hreath. She therefore holds the abdominal contraction while quickly taking in some more air through the open mouth, closing it again and continue to push. As soon as the contraction ceases, the mother must fully relax to be able to join into the next uterine contraction with renewed effort. This short rest period should be used to put the legs down and breathe as deeply as is comfortable.

As soon as the baby's head is ready to pass through the opening, the mother may have a strange sensation of smarting and will be asked to refrain from pushing as the head must come through slowly. It may be necessary to revert to panting breathing and the mother must be prepared to follow the instructions of her attendants. Once the head is born, the rest of the body will follow in a matter of minutes.

*Stage 3.*

There is usually a short interval between the birth of the baby and the delivery of the afterbirth. The mother should use this interval for full relaxation, stretching out her leg and deep breathing. She may be asked at the next uterine contraction to make again an expulsive effort.

## NINTH CLASS
### (35th Week of Pregnancy)

This final class should be used to make sure of breathing and muscle control during labour. It should primarily serve to answer any questions and remove any anxiety and doubt from the mother's mind.

These classes have been described at weekly intervals. The arrangement will however depend on local conditions.

Many women do better if they come weekly. This attendance never appears difficult to them or a trouble. There is enough material given in the preceding pages and the chapter which follows to fill weekly classes. The mothers, if primigravidae, have only imagination to draw upon, and need constant repetition of the main points of instruction if the picture is to become clear. Probably nine or ten classes is a good number, but even one or two are better than none, though obviously the best results are likely to occur with the greatest number of attendances.

# Chapter 4

## LACTATION

Breast feeding is the natural way to rear an infant. Emotion-
ally the new responsibility for the baby will be accepted much
more easily if the protective instinct present in every living
being can find an outlet by preparing the expectant mother for
the feeding problems of the baby. Breast feeding where
possible should be encouraged for many reasons, not the least
of them being the feeling of security it establishes in the baby
and the help it gives towards establishing a relationship
between the young mother and the baby. Artificial feeding
must however also be discussed antenatally with all its
problems. There may be psychological difficulties, or there
may be physical difficulties preventing a young mother from
feeding her baby. This is the reason why all the preparatory
work has been fitted into a seperate chapter. This should make
it easier to deal with the problem according to individual
requirements.

This class, after the exercises have been practised, is given
up to breast preparation. This instruction is frequently the
responsibility of the midwife. The mother should have a small
amount of oil (olive, castor, liquid paraffin, etc.) and a hand
towel. She should wear clothes which open up easily so that
both breasts can be treated. She may want to know first why
breast feeding is advocated and may need to be reassured
about her capability for doing it successfully.

The nipple must be inspected early in pregnancy and
treated if necessary if the mother wishes to breast feed.

*Positive facts concerning the baby*

1. There is an important relationship between the chemical
composition of mother's milk and the food with which the
foetus is nourished before birth, i.e. both are formed from the
mother's blood.

2. Breast milk contains a number of indefinite chemical
bodies which confer upon the infant the same kind of
immunity the mother herself possesses, therefore breast-fed

infants are probably less susceptible to disease than those artificially fed.

3. Breast milk undergoes certain progressive modifications concurrently with the development of the infant's stomach. Colostrum is present at birth, changing to milk in three days, and of progressively increasing strength.

4. Breast milk is free from harmful germs which may lurk where bottles, teats, etc., are used; in fact, it is always sterile.

5. Breast feeding is economical in time and money.

6. Breast milk is every baby's birthright. Nature has provided this food for his protection, and the mother who denies it to him without good reason is *stealing* from her baby.

7. Breast milk is always at the right temperature (i.e. body heat).

8. Breast milk does not sour or spoil.

9. Breast feeding helps to establish a relationship between mother and baby. It helps to give the baby a sense of security.

## Postive facts concerning the mother

Breast feeding is important for involution of the uterus and the restoration of the mother's figure.

*N.B.* The breasts should be supported by a good well-fitting uplift brassiere while pregnant and while nursing.

## Breast preparation practice

*Massage.* This is shown by the operator standing behind (using her hands as the mother will herself and then by the mother herself.

1. Both hands (one above the other) are placed above the breast resting on the chest; these are drawn apart (Fig. 24).

The mother is looking down on her own hands in these pictures.

1st *Movement.* The hands are placed one on top of the other above one breast and are then drawn apart with firm pressure.        Figure 24

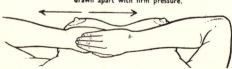

2. Both sweep down their own side of the breast, finger-tips downward (Fig. 25).

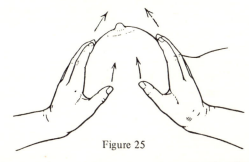

2nd Movement. The hands turn downward one on each side of the breast and, still pressing firmly, cup the breast approaching the areola and nipple.

Figure 25

3. Both cup the breast, fingers below, thumbs above, and draw the breast forward, allowing it to fall as the areola is reached (Fig 26).

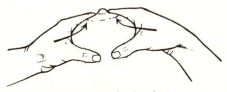

3rd Movement. As the encircling fingers and thumb reach the areola they glide off without touching it or the nipple.

The massage remains firm throughout.

Figure 26

This is repeated for five minutes, and the breast should then be flushed pink.

*Hand expression.* Again shown by the operator first and continued by the mother.

It is imagined that the baby is to be fed from say the left breast and will therefore be lying on the left arm. The right

48  *A Way To Natural Childbirth*

**I. By the mother herself.**

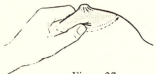

Figure 27

The fingers below and thumb above alternately compress and release the breast rather smartly and firmly (with a slight pressure backward into the breast at the same time)—their position is changed round the dotted line whenever milk ceases to flow.

In Fig. 25 it is assumed that the mother is looking down at her own right breast.

**II. By a helper (who can also use method I, standing behind mother).**

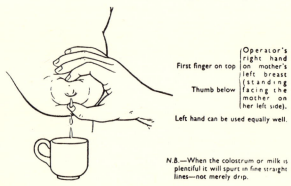

First finger on top

Thumb below

Operator's right hand on mother's left breast (standing facing the mother on her left side).

Left hand can be used equally well.

N.B.—When the colostrum or milk is plentiful it will spurt in fine straight lines—not merely drip.

Figure 28

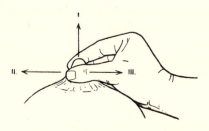

I. The nipple is pulled out by taking it between fingers and thumb first above and below and then on each side.

II. and III. The nipple is rolled between finger and thumb, finger going in direction II. and thumb in direction III., and then reversing.

Figure 29

hand will steer the breast and nipple towards the infant's mouth. It is pointed out that the baby should engulf areola and nipple and draw it to the back of the throat, and then by moving its lower *jaw* up and down exert the pressure which by suction draws the milk. If the left hand be used the index finger is placed *below* on the areola and the thumb *above* (Fig. 27) and a brisk pinching movement is performed (with a pressure inward at the same time). If the massage has been adequate fluid will soon *ooze* from the pores at the apex of the nipple (sometimes it may even *spurt out* in a fine jet). The beads of moisture or the jets should be counted and efforts made to add to the number of exits. (*N.B.* The other hand (right in this case) grasps the breast firmly (thumb above, fingers below). The grasping hand should be the outside one. The fluid which exudes may be colourless, straw-coloured, white, or bright yellow; it is called colostrum, and is the precursor of milk. Many mothers are afraid that they will not have milk, and the presence of this fluid is a great reassurance to them. Its relation to milk should be pointed out, also that it is an important food for the baby in its early days.

*Nipple drill.* The mother is shown how to draw out the nipple and roll it round to make it more supple and accustom it to use (Fig. 29). She is also advised three times a week for the last three weeks to put a small piece of lint with lanolin spread upon it over the nipple during sleep, washing and drying it thoroughly in the morning, and then doing the drill. This is to keep it supple and prevent dryness and cracking.

Some doctors disagree with this prac*t*ice and the advice of the medical attendant must therefore be sought.

# Chapter 5

## THE EVENTS OF LABOUR

Labour is always conducted by a medical man or woman or a midwife. It is therefore incumbent upon the physiotherapist who may attend labour to offer herself as someone extraneous to the delivery. Her place is at the head of the bed during the actual delivery, on the mother's left, in such a position that she never interferes with any routine (or unexpected) procedure. If she has established the right contact she may find herself constantly alone with the mother throughout the whole of the first stage (except for the routine events of examination, meals, and toilet). She is therefore free, by *consent* of those responsible, to help and advise the mother and move around as she wishes. She only needs to be with the mother when she is consulted.

Throughout labour the physiotherapist should bear in mind the acute sensitiveness of the woman in labour and her acute perception. Mothers will afterwards repeat remarks no one meant them to hear, they will detect glances unmeant for them, and sense any atmosphere of doubt, hesitation, and non-cooperation in a manner that has to be experienced to be believed. It is therefore most important to tell a 'trained' woman the truth in language she can understand and with deliberate intent to gain her cooperation and increase her confidence.

### Stage 1.

Most trained mothers will find no difficulty in moving about during the early part of this stage and then relaxing alone during contractions, usually any time up to three-fifths dilatation of the cervix. There are some who find it difficult after this and are grateful for massage in the form of firm back stroking. the majority, if they are going to find difficulty, find it at about four-fifths dilatation. Usually, however, firm stroking (Fig. 30) and encouragement are helpful. Inhalation analgesia is sometimes given at this time. In some cases the mother is given a sedative by mouth or injection *to help her to go on controlling her own relaxation.* The presence (or ability to be present at any moment) of an attendant is recognised as a necessity to women in labour, particularly from about three-fifths dilatation onwards. All through this stage quiet and peaceful surroundings are of the utmost help, and a husband who is as interested and well instructed as his wife is the best of all attendants. Many women show at the end of this stage a marked amnesia (unawareness of surroundings), and if relaxing well will doze or sleep between contractions, even *through* them. (On occasion, for instance, where labour is long or the early stages occur through the night, sedatives may be ordered to procure sleep).

As the mother becomes aware of her own sensations of the second stage approach, the physiotherapist can reinforce her impressions by knowledge. It should be pointed out here that a relaxed woman is often a surprisingly short time in passing from half to full dilatation, and this change should be estimated accurately, since neglecting to use the expulsive reflex causes unnecessary discomfort.

MASSAGE DURING THE FIRST STAGE OF LABOUR

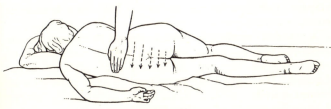

Figure 30

*Stage 2*

In the early part the physiotherapist can help in getting the expulsive effort well established. If the advance is slow and either the kneeling or squatting position is advocated, she can see that it is well done and effectual. As the child's head nears birth she can watch for the wishes of the doctor or midwife

and help to further them. Trained mothers have been coached
to expect the feeling of 'stretch' as the head dilates them fully,
and are not afraid of the sensation. They know they must
relax perfectly at this moment, and that soft panting breaths
with the mouth open will prevent expulsive movements if
these are not desired. They wish supremely to be present when
the child is born. A running commentary at this point from
the doctor or midwife is appreciated, and the mother will be
watching the appearance of the child and want to know when
head, arms, etc., are born. She likes to have it lifted out where
she can see it, and its cry is great happiness to her. She also
prefers to *ask* 'boy or girl' rather than be told.

Though the mother may have worked extremely hard in the
second stage and have felt and been extremely vociferous
about the overwhelming exhaustion she feels (always worse if
the night has been broken), the actual birth will be immediately followed by an intense feeling of physical well-being.
This, coupled with the mental delight, gives the mother an
impulse to sit up and grasp the child, and she expresses herself
as able to get up and resume her normal routine at once.

### Stage 3.

As soon as the cord is cut the child may be
wrapped and given to the mother to hold for a reasonable
length of time.

A trained mother is almost always interested in the
afterbirth. She is equally impressed by the relief which its
expulsion gives her and the feeling once again of a flat
abdomen. The size of her uterus (and its daily descent) is an
interest as well.

Once the delight of holding her baby has been experienced
and the baby taken to the cot, hunger and thirst (engendered
by the hard work) supervene, and it is customary to provide
the mother with a hot drink after the third stage is completed.
She is also quite ready to do real justice to the next meal when
it is ready. She dwells constantly on her experience and is a
transfigured woman.

As soon as the baby has been washed and put beside her in

its cot, the mother will lie holding the baby's hand or peeping at the child and find the greatest delight in this nearness. If it is suggested, she will be thrilled to have the baby to the breast soon after birth, and nothing is a better start for breast feeding than this.

## The husband

It has not been a general practice in the past for the husband to be present at his wife's labour. This is possibly understandable from a variety of angles, though not so readily if the desire of most married couples to share great experiences is considered. A woman who bears her child naturally is quite literally transfigured at the moment of its birth, and apart from the added joy she would have in sharing the child with its co-creator, it is the husband's right to take this share and witness his wife's attainment of motherhood if he wishes. Wherever husband and wife are equally well prepared and desire it, this would seem to be the procedure of the future.

# Chapter 6

## THE PUERPERIUM

The mother who has attended antenatal classes has a very good basis of knowledge for the restoration to function of her muscles. She will literally take this into her own hands if directed wisely and occasionally supervised. She feels so well that she is ready to start at once and go just as fast as her doctor will let her. It is well to explain that the uterus, though bulky at first, descends rapidly, and she can feel, if she wishes, this descent day by day. She should also be allowed to feel the separation between her recti muscles. This can best be done by lying quite flat and then lifting the head to look at the feet. The muscles will harden and the fingers can then press down into the space between them. The gap between them should close while in bed, but the stretched rectus sheath remains and only the muscle strength keeps the abdominal wall under control in the future. A further point of interest is to pass a tape measure round the abdomen at the level of the umbilicus and make a record of the decrease in inches as the abdominal muscles regain tone and the fat is absorbed. It is a point of pride with trained mothers that they get up able to wear their pre-pregnancy clothes.

Many doctors feel that the mother can begin her exercises and get out of bed straight away after a normal confinement. They keep her in bed for a short time however, as a safeguard against her overdoing things; once up, a woman finds it difficult to know where to stop, as there are likely to be so many demands upon her time and strength, and overstrain tends to react upon the milk supply and so ultimately to deprive the baby.

It is helpful to prepare a sheet of instructions such as the following for the mother's own use. The exercises can be followed individually or as classwork in a ward and given by the physiotherapist (see p. 60).

## INSTRUCTIONS TO MOTHERS AFTER CHILDBIRTH

A day or so after the birth of the baby it is both pleasant and a good thing to start simple exercises in bed. Breathing exercises and foot and leg movements have a good effect on the circulation and should be done while you are in bed. Gentle exercises will help the stretched abdominal and pelvic muscles to return to normal as quickly as possible. When getting out of bed, use this an an exercise—bend up knees, pull in abdominal muscles and swing legs over the edge of the bed. When standing—pull your abdominal muscles and buttock muscles tight and stretch up.

The following is a list of exercises which have been specially designed for you. With the approval of the doctor or midwife, they may be started the day after the baby is delivered. The exercises should be performed slowly and smoothly.

### First Day After Delivery

**Foot and leg muscle exercises and breathing**

*1. Lying with legs straight and slightly apart*
(a) Bend and stretch the ankles six times (Figs. 31 and 32).
(b) Bend and stretch the toes six times (Figs. 33 and 34).

FOOT EXERCISES

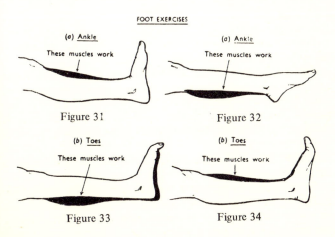

*(a)* Ankle

These muscles work

Figure 31

*(a)* Ankle

These muscles work

Figure 32

*(b)* Toes

These muscles work

Figure 33

*(b)* Toes

These muscles work

Figure 34

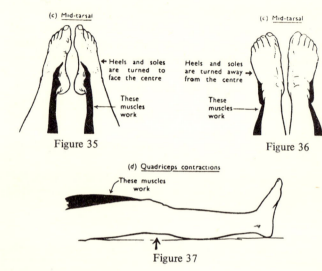

(c) Mid-tarsal

← Heels and soles are turned to face the centre

These muscles work

Figure 35

(c) Mid-tarsal

Heels and soles are turned away → from the centre

These muscles → work

Figure 36

(d) Quadriceps contractions

These muscles work

Figure 37

## 2. Lie on the back, knees bent.

(a) Breathe in, letting the abdomen swell out; breathe out and let it sink in (Fig. 6). Repeat three times.

Turn feet in and out (ankles bent up) six times (Figs. 35 and 36).
Tighten the muscles above the knee, six times (Fig. 37).

(b) Breathe in, expanding the ribs sideways and opening the inverted V under the breastbone, breathe out and let it sink back (Fig. 7). Repeat three times.

Repeat the above series of exercises three or four times a day during the first few days while you are still spending the greater part of the day in bed; when you are up and out of bed all day, omit the breathing exercises and do the foot and leg exercises when you have a chance to sit down and put your feet up.

*3. Lying with legs straight, if possible remove pillow.*

Pull your buttock and abdominal muscles tight and bend your feet up, making the whole body as straight as possible. Hold this position while counting six, then fully relax.

## Second Day After Delivery

Repeat the previous day's exercises and add Exercises 4 and 5.

**Exercise for the abdominal muscles**

*4. Lying on the back with knees bent, feet resting on the bed*

Tighten your seat muscles and pull in your abdomen so that your back is pressed against the bed. Hold this position while you count six, then relax. Repeat six times.

Practise this movement also when sitting out of bed.

**Contracting the pelvic floor muscles**

*5. Lying on the back with knees bent, feet resting on the bed*

Pull up the muscles through which the baby was born, thus tightening the opening of the birth passage (vagina). Hold the contraction for six counts, then relax. Repeat three times.

This muscle also closes the passage from the bladder. When learning this very important exercise, you can be sure that you are doing it correctly if you can stop the stream when you are passing water.

Practise this exercise also when sitting out of bed.

## Third Day After Delivery

Add Exercises 6 and 7 to the previous exercises.

**Contracting the waist muscles**

*6. Lie on the back with one knee bent and one straight*

Draw up the straight leg along the ground, making the waist line firm and much more curved inwards, push the leg back along the floor in the reverse direction. Do this with the other leg also. Repeat six times. (Fig. 12).

**Contracting the oblique abdominal muscles**

*7. Lying with knees bent and feet on the bed*

Draw in your abdominal muscles, reach across your body to place one hand on the opposite side of the bed on a level with the hip. Return to the starting position and repeat turning to the opposite side. Repeat three times.

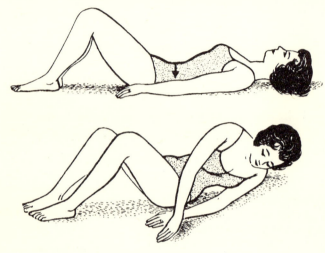

Figure 38

### Every Day

*Relaxation on the face.*

Put two pillows, one on top of the other, under your hips and lie flat face downwards over them (head preferably without a pillow and turned to one side), arms tucked under them and relaxed on the bed by the sides, feet on one pillow. Relax your whole body, and start your afternoon rest like this. If you sleep then, so much the better. The pillows under your hips are to keep your back from *hollowing* and so stretching your abdomen; they also leave room for your breasts and save the leaking of milk from pressure on them. It is wise to do this twice a day until the womb has returned to its normal size or until the doctor advises you that it is in a satisfactory position. Be sure that your bladder is empty and your bowels reasonably so before taking up the position.

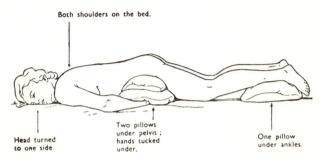

Both shoulders on the bed.

Head turned to one side

Two pillows under pelvis ; hands tucked under.

One pillow under ankles.

Figure 39

## Posture correction (Fig. 40)

Every day, lying with the legs straight, practice the four important postural points:

1. Contract the hip muscles.
2. Contract the lower abdomen.
3. Open out the ribs.
4. Straighten the neck against the bed.

This makes you stretch and grow taller.

Then relax and allow yourself to telescope.

Repeat this sitting up in bed (preferably with knees bent over the side), and as soon as you are allowed to stand up out of bed practise daily the correct standing position thus:

1. Get weight directly above instep and flatten *all* the toes on the floor.
2. Press the knees gently back.
3. Tighten the hip muscles.
4. Draw in the lower abdomen. Pelvic tilting
5. Open out the ribs.
6. Draw the head towards the ceiling, straightening back of the neck.

*N.B.* Arms should relax and shoulder drop naturally.

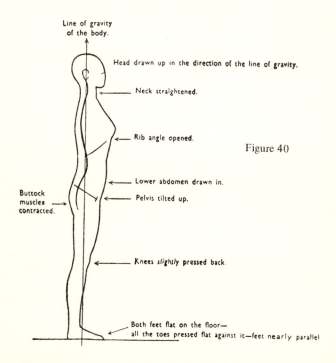

Line of gravity
of the body.

Head drawn up in the direction of the line of gravity.

Neck straightened.

Rib angle opened.

Figure 40

Lower abdomen drawn in.

Buttock
muscles ——→
contracted.

Pelvis tilted up.

Knees *slightly* pressed back

Both feet flat on the floor—
all the toes pressed flat against it—feet nearly parallel

Mothers should be given a period in the day when they can do these, and the room or ward be emptied of everyone else and their jobs, otherwise the mother finds it practically impossible to settle down to this most important restoration of her physical self.

## SUGGESTIONS FOR A WARD CLASS

Conditions differ in hospitals and it is therefore difficult to make rules. The general principles underlying these classes are however the same under most conditions.

1. The gaining of interest and cooperation from both the mother herself and from the nursing staff. It is therefore essential to discuss with the ward sister the most suitable time for the class. It should be a period which allows approximately

45 minutes for the class and, following this, as least 15 minutes of rest for the mother.

2. Procuring the greatest freedom of movement. (Drawing back curtains, removing pillows, turning down bedclothes, provision of washable 'pants' to go over the nightdress and free the legs etc.)

3. Giving a progression of exercises from day to day which builds towards the customary time for discharge. The exercises must be presented in such a way that the mother can easily understand the value for her own recovery and the value for regaining her previous figure.

4. Offering material on discharge for a daily continuation at home. She must be advised how she can build the essential exercises into her working day. The table is arranged in a suit-able order, having regard for the working of all relevant parts of the body, and at the same time for the progression day by day. The day upon which the mother joins in each exercise is there - fore stated; once a mother has joined in an exercise she continues with that every day and adds on the others daily.

The exercises are not illustrated as they are intended for use by the physiotherapist, to whom they will be quite familiar.

## TABLE OF EXERCISES

### First Day

**Lying with legs straight and slightly apart**
1. Bend and stretch ankles
**Crook lying**
2. Anterior abdominal breathing.
**Lying with legs apart**
3. Feet rolling round in circles in both directions.
**Crook lying**
4. Lateral costal breathing

### Second Day

**Repeat the earlier exercises and add:**
*Lying with legs apart*
5. Turn feet in and out (ankles bent up)

**Crook lying**
6. Abdominal and gluteal contractions
7. Pelvic floor contractions
**Sitting**
8. Shoulder circling for lactation when necessary
**Lying**
9. Complete postural contraction of quadriceps, glutei, abdominal muscles, back and shoulder muscles.
During this class and all the following classes all the exercises should be interspersed with the two breathing exercises taught on the first day.

### Third Day
**Repeat the earlier exercises and add:**
*Half croof lying*
10. One hip shortening—to be repeated on the other side.
11. One knee rolling over straight leg—to be repeated on the other side.

### Fourth Day
**Repeat the earlier exercises and add:**
*Crook lying*
12. Abdominal retraction combined with trunk rotation by placing one hand on the opposite side of the bed on a level with the hip. Practise rotation to alternate sides.

### Fifth Day
In shorts and getting out of bed, add the following exercises:
13. Postural correction in *(a)* standing, *(b)* sitting, and *(c)* walking.
14. Teach correct lifting.

### Sixth Day Until Discharge
The mothers take part in the full class.
After every class the mothers would spend at least 15 minutes in prone lying with a pillow under the hips.

# INSTRUCTIONS TO MOTHERS ON RETURNING HOME FROM THE HOSPITAL OR NURSING HOME OR ON GETTING UP AT HOME FOR THE GREATER PART OF THE DAY

A Home Exercise sheet should be handed to the mother containing the following information:

## Posture

A backward leaning posture sometimes becomes a habit during pregnancy and may persist after the baby is born. Transfer your weight from your heels more to the front of the ankle, tighten the buttock and lower abdominal muscles as in Exercise 4 and make yourself as tall as possible. Frequent conscious efforts to use these muscles will help to cultivate a good posture which will become a habit as the muscles grow stronger.

### Foot And Leg Muscle Exercises

Do any of these when you have a chance to sit down and put your feet up.

### Contracting The Pelvic Floor Muscles

Do this exercise in standing or sitting.

### Contracting The Waist Muscles

Do this exercise in standing.

### Contracting The Oblique Abdominal Muscles

Continue to do this exercise in the same way as previously learned. Every exercise should be repeated six times and the whole series continued for at least six weeks.

### Useful Advice About Your Back

A great deal of unnecessary backache can be avoided after childbirth if prolonged stooping is avoided as much as possible. Working surfaces should be at the correct height for the individual. An easy remedy when the sink is too low is to place the washing up bowl on a second upturned bowl. Avoid lifting heavy weights when you can, but on the occasion when you must lift something heavy, do not stoop over it with straight knees. Instead, bend the knees, hold the weight close to yourself and lift the weight by straightening hips and knees.

## Suggestions for Advanced Exercises

The previously described exercises represent essential basic exercises for restitution of muscle tone and good functional posture. If you are however interested after several weeks in slightly more strenuous exercises a few suggestions follow.

### Contracting the waist muscles

*On hands and knees.* Pull the abdomen up towards the spine, so that the back is completely flat, then swing the hips from side to side as if you were a dog wagging its tail, and turn your head every time to look at your 'tail' so that your waist line is well tucked in on the side to which you look. Repeat three times to each side and then rest. Repeat the whole series once more.

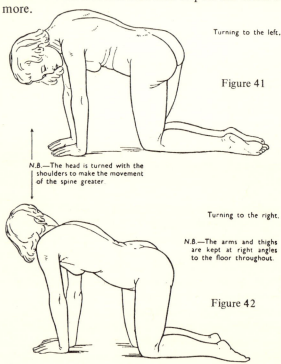

Turning to the left.

Figure 41

N.B.—The head is turned with the shoulders to make the movement of the spine greater.

Turning to the right.

N.B.—The arms and thighs are kept at right angles to the floor throughout.

Figure 42

## Contracting the oblique abdominal muscles

*On hands and knees* Swing the right arm under your body, then swing it sideways and upwards to the ceiling, turning your body and head to look up at it. Keep up this swing to alternate sides until you have completed three swings to each side. Then rest. Repeat the whole series once more.

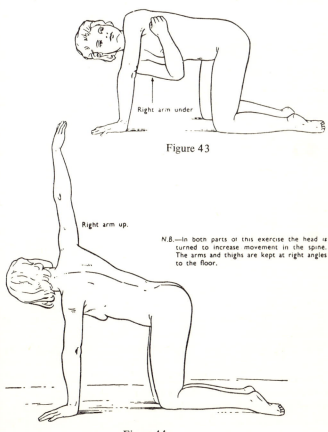

Right arm under

Figure 43

Right arm up.

N.B.—In both parts of this exercise the head is turned to increase movement in the spine. The arms and thighs are kept at right angles to the floor.

Figure 44

*Lying (knees bent, feet on the floor, and later feet off the floor) Arms spread out.* Roll both knees to one side until they touch the floor. Repeat to the other side. The abdomen must be well drawn in throughout the activity. When the abdominal muscles get stronger this exercise may be done with the feet off the floor. Repeat three times to each side then rest. Repeat the whole series once more.

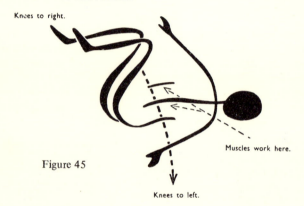

Knees to right.

Muscles work here.

Figure 45

Knees to left.

## LACTATION AND BREAST FEEDING

### Lactation and Breast Feeding

Lactation is the period after the birth of the child when the breasts secrete milk. As has been said already, colostrum precedes milk and can be demonstrated before the birth (often a number of weeks before), some mothers losing it spontaneously and some when hand expression of the breasts is attempted. Colostrum contains food for the baby, and since in a primipara it is usually not replaced by milk before the third postnatal day, the baby should be encouraged directly after a normal birth to suck and obtain this precursor of its later diet. In a multipara milk tends to be secreted much earlier, and the feeding of a second and subsequent child is therefore usually much easier at the beginning.

If the milk supply is tardy or congested much can be done to assist in successful breast feeding. This must be done early. Above all, engorgement must be avoided as it is always followed by deficiency. The massage and expression taught to the mothers during pregnancy can be used by them, preceded by contrast bathing, and supplemented by the following massage and exercises, according to the doctor's advice.

## Massage

One hand supporting the breast, the other kneads in small circles over the entire breast area, working systematically round the base first, and then spirally round to the areola. Done first with the palm or surfaces of the fingers, then with loose fist and backs of second row of phalanges (Fig. 46).

The whole should take five to ten minutes on each breast and be done twice daily an hour after a feed.

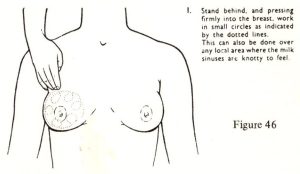

I.  Stand behind, and pressing firmly into the breast, work in small circles as indicated by the dotted lines. This can also be done over any local area where the milk sinuses are knotty to feel.

Figure 46

II.  Using the hand in the same way as Effleurage IV, the circular movement pressing into the breast tissue can be used

## Exercises

A few examples of exercises to be done between each feed are given.

*Sitting up in bed.* 1. Lift up the forearms by bending the elbows and squeeze the breasts together *very firmly* with the upper arms, gradually lifting the breasts upwards by lifting the arms thus bent (Fig. 47).

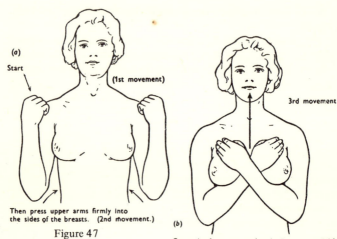

(a)
Start
(1st movement)

Then press upper arms firmly into
the sides of the breasts. (2nd movement.)

Figure 47

3rd movement

(b)

Cross the forearms under the breasts and lift
them, still crossed, in the direction of the arrow
until they are right above the head.
After a little way the breasts, having been lifted
up at first, will drop down again. (4th movement.)

Figure 48

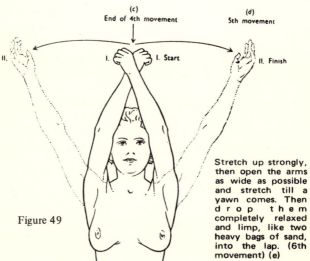

(c)
End of 4th movement

(d)
5th movement

II.          I.    I. Start                    II. Finish

Stretch up strongly,
then open the arms
as wide as possible
and stretch till a
yawn comes. Then
d r o p   t h e m
completely relaxed
and limp, like two
heavy bags of sand,
into the lap. (6th
movement) (e)

Figure 49

2. Go on lifting the arms and the breasts will drop suddenly (Fig 48).

3. Continue upwards with the arms, crossing the wrists, until they are straight above the head (Fig. 49).

4. Open the arms wide, reaching obliquely up to the corners of the room (Fig. 49).

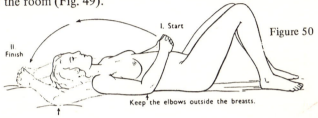

I. Start

Figure 50

II. Finish

Keep the elbows outside the breasts.

Press the elbows well into the bed.

5. Drop suddenly into the lap and start again. Do at least 12 times.

### Lying

*Knees bent, hands clasped on abdomen.* Take the arms with elbows bent above the head and lay the whole arm thus on the bed with firm pressure into the bed. Return the arms, stretching downwards as much as possible this time (Fig. 50).

### Sitting

*Knees bent, one hand resting on the bed.* Bend the other arm across in front above the resting hand, then take it slowly and strongly out to its own side at shoulder height, turning the palm gradually to look upward and going as far backward with it as possible. Repeat (after 12 times) with the other arm (Fig. 51).

Both the lying and the sitting exercises should be done 12 times in all at first and increased daily until the milk supply is adequate.

### Contrast Bathing

Two bowls and two cloths (baby's nappies will do if scrupulously clean):

1. Containing ice-cold water and cloth.

2. Containing the hottest water the mother can tolerate. (*N.B.* Keep a can of boiling water handy for refills.)

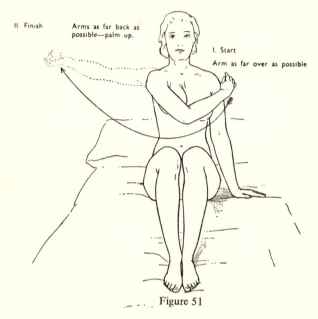

II. Finish  Arms as far back as possible—palm up.

I. Start

Arm as far over as possible

Figure 51

Use each bowl alternately, splashing one breast at a time for five minutes with hot water, then one minute with cold water. Repeat three times starting and ending with hot water. Dry vigorously with a rough towel, rubbing towards the nipple all the time. Pat the nipple dry, but do not rub it.

Do twice daily immediately before the massage.

### Conditions Conducive to Successful Feeding after the Mother has been thus Educated to have Confidence in Herself

(She should know that there can never be a true substitute for breast milk)

*Place.* The mother's own room or nursery, mother and child being *alone*. They have to learn to know one another. If in a hospital ward there should be cubicles, with curtains to draw, ideally. Many mothers are selfconscious and ashamed if their babies are not all they should be at once. Patience is an essential.

*Help.* This should always be available both during the lying-in period *and at home after.* If needed it should be given by an expert, and preferably the same person all the time.

*Food.* This must be adequate in quality and quantity, and contain liberal drinks of water (a glass every feed is a good rule).

*Quality.* Proteins, fats, and carbohydrates must all be present in correct proportions, and an ample supply of vegetables and fruit (uncooked as well as cooked) and fresh milk. All the vitamins are of paramount importance.

*Quantity.* The mother *must* satisfy her hunger thoroughly and, particularly if the baby is big and hungry, she may need extra (nourishing) food such as milk drinks between meals.

*Worry. Freedom from worry of any kind is very important.* This is where the husband and friends can be so helpful.

*Rest. An afternoon rest* should be taken to make up for the shorter and possibly interrupted night necessitated by feeding the baby, during the period of establishing a feeding routine.

## Chapter 7

## The Mothers have their Say

Nothing can be more convincing as proof of the value of any method than the spoken or written opinions of those who have put it into practice. Hearsay, generally of a frightening nature, is all that an expectant mother has to guide her in her first experience of childbirth. That is why the accounts written by women who have actually experienced joy and happiness in their first childbirth are so valuable to all who wish to learn. The *description* of sensations, though it can never equal the actual *experience* of them, can go a very long way towards it.

This book, so far, has concerned itself with setting out a method of following certain now well established principles. At this point it deviates to allow the mothers who have tried that method to say what they think,

Extracts have been selected from nearly 200 accounts (all first experiences except the few specially noted), and have been grouped into a sequence showing the events of labour. The sub-headings employed are based upon those laid down by Dr Grantly Dick Read (see Bibliography, No. 18).

Sub-headings:
1. Announcement.
2. Preparation Classes.
3. First Stage.
4. Transition from First to Second.
5. Second Stage.
6. Third Stage.
7. In Retrospect.

### 1. Announcement

*Mrs B.* 'Well, another dear little son (Michael John), and what a grand experience this time more than ever. It's going to be difficult to write this without appearing to write a personally boastful missive.'

## 2. The Preparation Classes

*Mrs J.* 'Before I started attending the classes my knowledge of the actual course of a birth was perfunctory. I looked forward to the mysterious horrors of labour as a necessary evil, and one of the most tremendous benefits I derived from the classes was the knowledge and confidence implanted by the teachers.'

*Mrs K.* 'During the nine months previous to the baby's birth I had continually "worried" because my elder sister had had a very "bad time" with both her first and second babies, as she was in labour 72 hours and she had to have forceps.

'But after my baby's birth I did not consider it an ordeal at all, and only once was I afraid when the physiotherapist said that she was going to phone and I did not like the idea of being left alone.'

*Mrs L.* 'I enjoyed the classes for three reasons: Firstly, for the exercises themselves, especially because the reason for each one was so carefully explained to us. Secondly, for the jolly fellowship with the other members. Thirdly, and most of all, for the counsel and advice the physiotherapist constantly gave us out of her own experience. We besieged her with questions on every aspect of pregnancy, childbirth, and mothercraft, and she always gave us a full and satisfying answer. If I may say so, the fact that she herself was a mother made her completely "approachable," and her enthusiasm and intense interest were infectious, and she never made any of us feel we were "just another case". She gave us such a vivid detailed account of labour that I could picture it almost as well as if I had been through it before, and this of course was an enormous help.

'I had a very happy pregnancy, due, I believe, to physical well-being and mental confidence. My friends constantly commented on my extreme fitness. I am 34, had no proper sex education, have a spinal curvature, and am subject to low blood pressure. Yet this training dispelled any doubts or fears I had, and I felt very confident. I was particularly glad to know that the physiotherapist was willing to be with us during labour, for the prospect of being left alone at all would have appalled me I'm afraid.'

*Mrs B. 1. Attitude to childbirth before pregnancy.* 'Before becoming pregnant myself my attitude was one of awe, regarding the phenomenon as something wonderful yet full of unpredictable dangers and unspoken agony. My knowledge of the actual process of childbirth was practically *nil.*

*2. Attitude early in pregnancy.* 'I was delighted to find that I was to have a child, but felt that I was to face something unknown, rather terrible, that would possibly take my life. (Two of my friends had died in childbirth).

'I decided myself that during labour I would try to lie quite still, letting the pains, the nurses, and the doctor do the job. Thus I anticipated only passive not active co-operation.

'I was definitely afraid of:

(a) The inevitable loss of personal dignity attached to labour.

(b) The "Mess"

*3. Attitude after attending the classes.* I soon began to feel an eagerness to perform the job we were being trained for and lost all the stupid fear of the attitudes to be assumed in labour, developing gradually an objective approach in place of the purely subjective and emotional one. I was also grateful for the many little hints as to what to expect, as thereby fears were allayed which might have caused serious inhibitions at the time, e.g. to expect cramps, shiverings, etc. The detailed knowledge of the process of labour removed all fears of the unknown which had been present.'

*Mrs L.* 'By the time the baby was due I was quite sure that I could carry through a natural birth successfully, and was determined not on any account to be given any "dope." I wanted to see the child born, to hear his first cry, and welcome him in my arms within a few minutes, and I shall always be grateful that I experienced all these joys.

'When I was attending the classes I soon realised how little I really knew about the details of childbirth before. And I think this thoroughness was of great value. For instance, when I vomited during labour and when I had a violent attack of shivering I didn't worry a bit, as I immediately remembered that the physiotherapist had warned us it might happen and told us not to let it bother us.'

*Mrs H.* 'The relaxation classes proved a great help to me both before the actual labour and during labour. I had no knowledge of childbirth or of the various parts of the body and their action during pregnancy. This was explained, and a good few old-fashioned theories were squashed which would have been worrying if not.'

*Mrs B.* 'I thoroughly enjoyed the company and behaviour of other expectant mothers, and what a lovely time we had discussing our very minor ailments. I should very much like to meet those mothers and babies twelve months hence.'

*Mrs M.* *'Mental reaction to childbirth before marriage.* Definitely one of fear due to ignorance. (In my day at college we did not touch the subject.) The knowledge that my sister's first labour was long and difficult and her second child was still-born.'

### First Stage

*Exhilaration*

*Mrs L.* 'I left home very joyfully, and one of the best tributes is that my husband was completely confident too. Considering I was in labour all day Sunday till 10.45 p.m., and my husband, a minister, carried through a heavy programme of services without people even suspecting I had started is worth noting.'

*Mrs L.* 'First came a slight show and with it a great feeling of joy and excitement that at last my baby was starting on the last part of his journey into the world. . . ' (Membranes then ruptured.)

### Soberness

*Mrs L.* 'Then came the midnight journey to the nursing home with all the baby's things, the first sight of my room, and the waiting for the first contraction. Perhaps, too, there was a feeling of slight apprehension of the coming hours which were full of not the unknown, but better expressed—the unexperienced.'

*Mrs J.* (second baby) 'I arrived here at about 5 p.m., and after the usual toileting I got to work in earnest about 6 p.m. Dr R. came to see me very shortly after, and everything was very satisfactory. At this point I must say that I was completely confident and perfectly happy. From then on I was able to get on with my relaxing undisturbed, and apart from sister looking in now and again was left in peace until Dr R. came in at 10 p.m. I believe I rather surprised him by being almost five fingers dilated. I know I surprised sister; I don't think she thought I was having real contractions. Dr R. ruptured the membranes, and from then on everything went full-speed ahead.

'In comparison I can say that I had accomplished in four hours what had previously taken me over forty. I was still complete mistress of the situation. A great tribute to the powers of relaxation.'

*Mrs L.* 'I felt too "lazy" to walk about and lay on the bed most of the day, and we chatted about all sorts of things in between contractions. I found that the more completely I relaxed the better it was, in fact I enjoyed using at last what we had been taught to practise for so long, and the physiotherapist massaged my back.

'The day held plenty of humour, as when my meals were solemnly served to me in the labour ward, and I felt a humbug being there at all. The doctor and the matron came in from time to time to note progress. There was another girl in the nursing home in the first stage, and I used to greet the matron with, "Who is winning?" and "What is the score this time?" '

*Mrs V.* 'I found that the best way to meet the contractions at this point was to imagine that the undulations of the pain were a range of mountains, up and down the ever-increasing heights of which I bore myself on my own breath. This, of course, was the practice of the deep breathing we had been taught. It was invaluable. The last gloriously smooth slide down the last slope into the most wonderful peace that can ever be experienced was ample reward for the sustained effort of "mountaineering," and gave something to look forward to as the contractions recurred. I think that this wonderful sense of peace can be felt only by a person in full control of her labour.

'I also found that, as this stage advanced, I could brook no interference with the contractions, and when someone came to see me I would excuse myself from the conversation whenever one occurred. It was towards the end of this stage that I so much appreciated the gentleness and the "niceness to look at" of my physiotherapy attendant. The rather determined cheerfulness of the nurse I found irksome and unnecessary. I wanted only to practise the relaxation the whole time, finding it easier to enter the contractions fully relaxed if I maintained that attitude throughout.'

*Mrs B.* 'I remember distinctly thinking, as I lay there, how perfectly *normal* I felt in between each contraction. I still marvel that I had no fear; my whole energies, mental and physical, seemed to be concentrated on a job in a world of its own.

'I was examined by a doctor who said it would be "Some hours". Nurses kept asking me, "Was I getting any pains." and I kept saying "No". In retrospect it seems almost humorous that I didn't realise that the contractions I was getting *were* the so-called "pains"! When I told the patient in the next bed that I was getting these every quarter of an hour *she* sent for the nurse again, who examined me and told me to walk to the labour ward.'

*Mrs B.* 'I *really* started to have *definite* and *regular* contractions (but *not* severe) every ten minutes at 12. I did relax for these, but they didn't require much effort.

'*Dr B.* came to see me at 12.45 and was *very* nice, and it *thrilled* me and greatly encouraged me too, I might say, to see *how* impressed he was by my relaxing and the impression it was having on the midwives here.

'During my first-stage contractions one midwife came to me and said, "I think we'll have to send you to the "green" to do some shopping to *get going!*" I thought "I'm going" all right but really, you know, one doesn't like to keep saying things like that. There's absolutely no doubt but that until you actually *show* them your conduct in labour *throughout* they think it's some sort of cult. You see it was only when I got to second stage that they *really* believed I'd been in first.'

### An unusual experiment

'Being even calmer than last time and understanding what stage I'd got to this time so much more, I thought I'd really give the relaxation a good trial for one or two contractions, and for about two contractions I tried gripping the rail of the bed in the "orthodox" way. Phew! it was *awful,* the harder you gripped the more it felt as if you were gripping your own inside. I only had the moral courage to try it about twice.'

### Need for companionship

*Mrs H.* 'The contractions became quite severe at 3 p.m., but with the help of the physiotherapist I managed to relax, and the deep breathing worked wonders when I got it right. Although there was some pain, it was bearable. All the time I felt cheerful and never that it was too much for me. Fear never entered my head.'

*Mrs V.* 'During the afternoon I must have slept for a while as when I wakened I was examined and told that my baby's head was showing and he would be born in less than half an hour's time. This was a very pleasant surprise for me as I realised that the dilatation of my vervix, a stage which I believed would be painful, had taken place without me even being aware of it. My mind was so fully occupied with wondering if the baby would be a little boy, which I so much wanted, and what he would be like that it only seemed a few minutes before he was born.'

### 4. Transition from First to Second Stage—Four-Fifths to Full Dilatation

*Demand for kindly but firm sympathy and assistance.*

*Mrs L.* 'And I regret to say I went "all to pieces"! I became irritable with the poor physiotherapist and said all sorts of silly things when we were alone in the labour ward such as, "Oh, I can't go on, I'm utterly done up," "Let me go to sleep, I'm so tired." I think I wanted to hear her say all the encouraging things she did say in reply. And I mention that I was artful enough to misbehave when we were alone, as I honestly don't believe I ever meant to be given anything, even in my worst moments of weariness. She was splendid, but was probably far more respectful than I deserved. You know me better than she does. I think if you had been there you would have been stricter, given me a "good ticking off," or threatened to march out and leave me to it, or found some means or other of shaking me to my senses.'

*Onset of amnesia.*

*Mrs D.* 'I can't remember whether there was anyone in the ward with me; things might have been happening, but I wouldn't have noticed; I felt I couldn't be bothered to make the effort, even to open my eyes. I vaguely heard Mr C.'s name mentioned, then Mr C.'s voice said my name. I don't know whether I answered; I felt I couldn't be bothered to do anything. Then I heard you say my name and told you when I wanted my back rubbing. What a relief that rubbing was. I felt that I wanted to push hard, and it was difficult not to. I remembered how to stop by panting hard.'

*Early expulsive efforts commencing*

*Mrs P.* 'At one stage I was suddenly very sick. Strangely

enough this was a great relief to me. I remembered your words on the subject of being sick between the first and second stages, and it was a great comfort to know that at last I could get down to work.'

### Conflict: 'confidence v. fear'

Dr A. 'I was then left alone until 9.55, and from about 9.15 to 9.55 relaxation became almost impossible. I'm afraid I did not recognise that this was the end of the first stage and I began to get afraid—if the contractions were going to get worse, what were they going to be like? I think the discomfort at this stage was severe enough to be called pain.'

### Early expulsive efforts commencing

'At 9.55 I could not keep up the regular breathing during contractions and held my breath, only to find that I wanted to push. The contractions were still every four minutes and I had no hicoughing, vomiting, shivering, or cramp, so I think I can be excused for not recognising the second stage earlier.'

### Confidence and relaxation after gaining the upper hand lead to early expulsive efforts

Mrs B. (second baby) 'From 1 to 2 I had them every five minutes, but not any more severe. From 2 to 2.45 they became nearer and nearer together. Sister came to look at me—and tucked me in! I thought secretly, "There's not much point in tucking me in, my dear, I'm off to the labour ward at any moment," but she obviously thought, "Well, she's no trouble, but relaxation isn't getting her very far!" However, with only two more contractions I began to feel that diaphragm business going the wrong way and the feeling of heaving.

'After only *two* I thought, "well, I shall just *have* to bear down" and called the nurse. She said, "I don't think you're ready, you know, but come across to the labour ward." (Baby born half an hour later.)

*Conflict: confidence and relaxation v fear and tension*

Mrs L. 'I was shortly to reach the stage in my labour which I consider was the most difficult to overcome, namely, the period which later proved to be the end of the first stage. I was at first rather light-headed and made rather stupid remarks, and then I became despondent, tired and, to be quite truthful, I did not like it. Had I realised then that the second stage was so near, things would have been easier, but I was told "There is only three fingers dilatation, it may take a long time yet." I shall know in future that incomplete dilatation does not necessarily imply that the second stage is not imminent, for I was soon to have a violent attack of shivering and shaking, and soon after the catch in the breath and desire to push and empty my bowels every time a contraction came, which was by now almost continuously.

'I was told to push down, and owing to my lack of confidence I only half-pushed, which meant that I felt considerable pain, but I soon made myself push with all my strength only to find that it did not hurt at all.'

*Second state amnesia, impatience and frustration, mental and physical exhaustion.*

'Just before I gained this confidence, however, my mind became confused. I was only half-aware of the people in the room. I desperately wanted to give the whole thing up for a while and come back to it after a long sleep. My advice to mothers at this stage would be, do *not* give in; this feeling is the sign that your baby will soon be born.

'In my case my son was born a short while later after I had given a few colossal pushes down which seemed to fill my anus.'

## 5. Second Stage. Hard Work Enjoyed

*Mental alertness*

Dr A. 'From now on it became plain sailing though very hard work. I rang for the nurse, who was very surprised when a P.R. confirmed that I was in the second stage. She sent for Dr S. I think I used the contractions well, and certainly rested well between them, though I never had the amnesia that is described.' (She *did*, because she told the sister how to deliver the baby, and does not remember this.)

'I was delivered at 11.10 p.m. in the *L* lateral position and saw the baby's head while the body was still inside me, and saw the rest of the delivery. It was most thrilling. I got a slight laceration of the vaginal mucosa of which I am ashamed, because I cannot have been completely relaxed, but this did not need suturing.'

### Physical signs of expulsive efforts

Mrs D. 'They let my husband in while the second state contractions were just beginning, and he, *knowing all about it,* said afterwards that if he hadn't known he would have thought me to be in great pain because I went very red in the face and the veins in my neck stood out. He didn't stay long, as things seemed to be moving so fast, but was back within a quarter of an hour of Anne's birth, so that we were able to share the feeling of elation.'

*Sense of accomplishment.* 'I didn't find the first stage bad at all, and really enjoyed the second stage. *It was a very satisfying experience altogether, and after it was over I felt I wanted to tell the world.'*

### Impatience and frustration exasperation threatens confidence

Mrs N. 'All sensation was in the rectum till just before crowning; it was a great help to be told the baby's head was coming down well as there was no sensation whatever that I was moving him. I remember feeling my abdomen anxiously with my hands to see if it was less bulgy. Bearing down movements were most exhausting and tiring, very uncomfortable but not painful. It was such hard work I wondered if I should have enough energy for the next one. Never sweated so much before. I remember saying, "This is awful!" Great relief when doctor and specialist came back. Was fully aware of what was happening. That first lusty cry was wonderful to hear; it gave such a feeling of elation and relief at success.'

*Amnesia between contractions*
  *Mrs D.* 'I certainly felt "dopey" throughout the second stage, and can't imagine why any patient would *want* an anaesthetic for this delivery. I can, however, see that if a patient has not been trained to hold her pushing and has not done any exercises to increase the elasticity of the muscles of her birth canal, then an anaesthetic would lessen the likelihood of a tear, but why not do the exercises and "be there" when your baby is born? I wouldn't have missed the experience for anything.'

  *Mrs P.* 'Once the "pushing" became easier I felt much happier. I found I could hold my breath throughout each contraction, and having had "rehearsals" at the classes was a tremendous help. I felt really "dopey" between contractions, and found I had to pull myself together quite firmly to get down to work when a contraction came on, as the "dopey" feeling was such a blissful comfort.'

*Training prevents fear and tension at the moment of birth, removing the need for analgesia and giving the mother her supreme experience. ·*
  'I think it was at this stage that the preparation we had had in the classes was the greatest help. I knew it wouldn't be much longer by the increased bustle in the labour ward and the encouraging note of anticipation and expectancy in people's voices. I kept telling myself, "Soon it will feel as though I'm going to split, but I mustn't let that worry me as it's a perfectly normal feeling." And when the feeling *did* come I felt quite triumphant and smug because I had been ready for it! I remember thinking in a detached kind of way, "They're quite right, it doesn't *hurt*." It just feels rather odd and uncomfortable, and it could be very, very frightening if you weren't ready for it.'

*Incredulity and facinated wonder*
  'I was just getting ready to be told to go over on to my side and start panting when the head was born. I had my eyes shut

and it gave me quite a shock as I wasn't expecting it until a good bit later. Then everything happened quickly. I saw the baby appear with the next contraction (or at least I saw *something*, but as I had taken off my spectacles when I started to work properly everything was a little hazy!). Two voices said in chorus, "It's a boy," and immediately there was a lusty and very bad-tempered sounding cry. Quite the most wonderful noise I'd heard in ages! I heard myself go all sentimental and slushy, which must have sounded *quite* ridiculous. But it was the most gorgeous feeling.'

### The explosion of an erroneous idea

*Mrs B.* 'Thank you for the unexpected pleasure of actually seeing my Susan born. I had never contemplated this possibility before hearing your lectures, taking it quite for granted that I should be under an anaesthetic.'

### Enchantment

*Mrs J.* (second baby) 'Then at last I was allowed to give the final little push and there was my lovely daughter squirming by my thigh. That was certainly something which came up to and surpassed everything which has ever been written about it. And all this without a single stitch. My old scar stood the strain after all. Dr R's skilful delivery plus relaxation and exercise must surely be responsible for this.'

### Mental alertness

*Mrs G.* (second baby; first was a forceps and mother unconscious under anaesthetic when it was born): 'When the head was "crowned" the relief was indescribable, and it was a most extraordinary experience to be able to look down and see the head there, with the baby's body still kicking inside. I think she cried at this stage. I had found it very interesting all through this last part to be able to look down in between contractions and see how things were going.'

### Fundamental primitive self appearing

*Mrs L.* 'I began having the real second stage contractions, and they were exactly as you had described them to us in the class. I was tremendously pleased to feel this sudden change, even though they were extremely strong and preceded by searing backache. I realised that this really was where it was up to me, and enjoyed the experience of hard cooperative work. Immediately there flashed into my mind all that you had stressed about great care at this point to avoid a tear. I could only avoid pushing by the rapid panting. I was so very glad I knew what to do. It would have been too late for anyone to tell me how to do it then. I'm afraid, in spite of all my care, I had to have one stitch. The humour of the situation suddenly returned, and when these contractions came (in rapid succession) I fairly shouted at matron, "It's coming on, shall I push or pant?" which became reduced to "Push or Pant? Push or pant?" I was enjoying myself at last, and the way in which I had suddenly become such an urgent, demanding creature amused me. If the whole of the second stage had been like this it would have been grand. It was exactly as you had described it to us.'

### Fascinated wonder

'The actual pushing out of the child was marvellous; a thrilling experience. I think I knew it was a boy as soon as the others did, and I was fascinated to see him struggling and crying there. I suppose all mothers ask the question I did, "Is he all right?" and the answer completed my sense of joy.

'All tiredness fled, never to return. I had a detached interest in the tying of the cord and "mopping-up operations." I felt completely normal immediately after the birth and have done so ever since. I was so pleased about this and somehow surprised, in spite of all the teaching about childbirth being a natural function!'

*Mrs. B.* (second baby) 'Another thing I had this time that I didn't have before was the much talked-of stretching feeling in second stage as if you're goint to burst. Although at heart I didn't really think one could, I do think that if you hadn't that very morning said to me, "Now do remember that if you do have that feeling, still push your hardest and it won't hurt!" I might have slipped up. . .For the push for the head I felt as if I were on fire round there. I suppose it was the smart of the stretch. I don't know; it certainly wasn't painful.'

*Mrs L.* 'I had no anaesthetic during my confinement and I certainly did not require one, although it was offered me and I refused it; and I am very glad I did, as I would not have missed the actual birth of my daughter for anything at all. In my opinion mothers who are given an anaesthetic at the time of the actual birth of their babies are robbed of that feeling of complete achievement and the crowning of all their efforts. It is the high-light of the whole nine months' waiting and the confinement itself.'

*Mrs S.* 'Two contractions were wasted by my keeping my mouth open to grunt and pant instead of closing my mouth and pushing. One of the nurses tried to make me have gas, but sister explained that she didn't think I should want it as I was a relaxation patient. It was cold and I felt shivery, but not the uncontrolled shuddering I had expected. I had no hiccoughing. They partly shaved and cleaned me between the next two contractions and real pushes, while I held my own leg up. Sister asked me if I wanted a whiff. I said, "No, unless I did not behave as she wanted at the critical period, in which case I would have it to prevent a tear." She asked me to pant when she told me. Then followed three really good pushes with sustained pushing and breathing; I could feel the terrific stretching. During pushes I had my head bent forward on to my chest where I was hugging a hot bottle, my other hand held my leg up. My husband came in and they told him where he could find a mask.

'11.40 a.m. Sister said the head was crowned. I did not feel pain at all while the rest of the head was born, just the moving forward of a large object. Dr R. Arrived and watched sister. There was more stretching as the shoulders were born. I panted and felt the infant being gently helped to come out. M. told me it was a boy. I felt him kicking my buttocks. I felt as though pints of water were pouring out. I saw him lying at the foot of the bed. The sister and Dr R. then looked to see if I had any tears, but I hadn't.'

*Enchantment*

Mrs. L. 'The terrific stretching feeling which is apparent when the head comes through did not frighten me as, thanks to prenatal classes, I knew it meant only a matter of minutes before the most wonderful and most joyous moment of all—the *actual moment* of my little son's birth. He was born, the joy was indescribable, his first little cry assured me he was alive and immediately my body was peaceful.'

## 6. Third Stage

*Satisfying sense of accomplishment.*

Mrs. B. 'After the birth a pleasant lassitude crept over me, in fact I couldn't think of anything except to look at Susan and say, "Well, fancy that." The placenta reminded me exactly of "lights"!'

Mrs M. *'Third stage:* I don't know how long this took. The placenta came away with very little bleeding, and sister was delighted at the way the uterus went hard quickly like a cricket ball.'

Mrs P. 'I believe the third stage lasted ten minutes—it seemed like two! I asked for the afterbirth to be held up for me to see; a very odd sight!'

*Restitution. (Welcome refreshment noted in all three of these)*

'Afterwards I felt very happy, very interested in a cup of tea, and very conscious of my new status of "mother". The world had changed for me, and from then on must become a fuller place and I more aware of its possibilities and its responsibilities.'

Mrs. L. 'The babe was bathed before he was handed to me,

and I held him in my arms for a few moments. I felt a quiet gladness as I welcomed "John," and realised that here at long last was the child of our dreams. I did not feel very emotional in the ordinary sense, but a very deep contentment. This may have been due to the small room being full of very busy people, and I found myself thinking, "This must be a very ordinary daily job to them though so important to me!"

'When I was settled in my room I sat up and had tea and bread and butter, and felt so well and wideawake, though it must have been midnight. When they put John in a cot across the room I remember reminding myself that I mustn't jump out of bed and have a look at him, I felt so fit I easily could have done so in an absentminded moment!'

*Mrs S.* '12.15 p.m. The placenta was born. There was no pain, only a slight return of the 'nagging period pain.' I held the bathed infant, who certainly looked healthy enough but not very handsome with his head not recovered from the moulding process and nose completely flattened like a negro. He had no wrinkles on his face and had a rosy complexion.

'12.30 p.m. We all had a cup of tea, and I was washed and changed into clean things, which made me feel grand.

12.50 p.m. Two nurses carried me into the bedroom.

1.10 p.m. I sat up in bed and ate stew and sprouts, with milk pudding and rhubarb to follow.

2 p.m. I had Christopher to the breasts and he sucked a tiny bit. I just lay and dozed all afternoon feeling grand.

'On Sunday I astonished everyone by moving my bowels without a laxative, and have managed it ever since, practising religiously abdominal and pelvic contractions.

'In spite of the worry before the birth and the interruption of relaxation, I am terribly thankful that I had been to all the classes and had every detail explained and every possible stage gone into thoroughly, so I knew what to expect and all the ways and means of preventing unnecessary pain at my disposal. I have no stiffness of joints so far as I can find out by moving about in bed, and I don't mind in the least the thought of going through it all again.'

## 7. In Retrospect

*Mrs L.* 'I am sure that if I could go through exactly the same experience again I would do a lot better! I look forward to having my next baby, and shall certainly practise relaxation again and the exercises, and I am quite determined to have the rest of our family in this natural way.'

*Mrs N.* 'I was very pleased about everything, and I shall always look upon the birth of my daughter as a new experience rather than something I want to forget.'

*Mrs O.* 'Well, I had a grand confinement, thanks to the instruction I have had from the exercise class, and all I can say to those left in the March class awaiting their babies' arrival is carry on with the exercises up to the end and you will be well rewarded by an easy birth of your baby.'

*Mrs G.* (second child) 'One of the nice things about this method of childbirth is that the memory of it is definitely a *pleasant* one, and I was the only one in the ward who was honestly able to say after a week, that provided I had the strength I would not in the least mind going through it again at once.

'Another thing I notice is that I somehow feel this child is much more my own since I took such part in her un-ceremonious arrival instead of having her brought to me hours after her actual birth looking as though she might have arrived by post.'

*Mrs A.* (a home confinement) 'I had a very easy con-finement and everything went very smoothly and easily. According to the nurse and doctor, "If everyone did as well as you we'd be able to retire." I feel very well, and the baby is beautiful. Sally Anne is her name. I know that most of the ease and all my confidence was the result of attenting the classes. I had no qualms and felt as though I knew what to do. . . . Before I came to the classes the whole business seemed rather terrifying and dangerous, and yet when the baby was coming I felt perfectly happy and quite unapprehensive.'

*Mrs G.* (second baby) 'It is a little difficult to compare this birth with the previous one, as I had been so doped I remember very little. The matron, who had been present at the first and delivered the second, said that the former was a forceps delivery and the second would have been had I not been following the relaxation method. I don't think I had any less pain in the first, and it seemed to be of a more hopeless nature. *Pain when one is semiconscious seems more unpleasant than when one is fully conscious,* and the tablets I had during the first labour did not really help much. The difference afterwards (with the relaxation method) is very marked. . . . I could never have written all this description (five closely covered pages) three days after the birth of my first child. My husband comments how much better I am this time.'

*Mrs M.* 'I have no bitter or agonising thoughts regarding my labour. I am perfectly confident that next time will be even better. I find myself trying to explain to everybody I meet the benefits obtained from antenatal exercises and relaxation. I feel I would like to shout it from the roof-tops. And my baby is so good; he sleeps every minute that he isn't feeding.'

*Mrs P.* 'I really can't tell you how grateful I am to all who made these classes possible; not only during labour did they prove invaluable but all through pregnancy; I'm sure I shouldn't have felt so confident and cheerful about everything during the months of waiting, and my whole outlook would have been totally different. I'm certain this calmness has made a difference to the baby's health, he seems so placid and contented. A note of interest: A number of people who have seen me feeding Christopher have said they have never seen a baby relax so perfectly once he has started to suck. Do you think this has anything to do with relaxation practices while I was carrying him?'

*Mrs A.* 'I have felt so incredibly well since baby's birth that

I feel I want to say only that it was all wonderful. I loved every minute of it, and am simply longing now for the advent of my four sons.'

*Mrs B.* (second baby) 'I cannot emphasise too fully the value of having someone with the mother in labour to help her carry out the exercises she has been taught. If she knows what she has to do, her mind immediately responds to the voice of someone telling her what to do. At the final stages she may be physically incapable of responding, but her mind, knowing what to do, seems to act at once and the body immediately does what is necessary. That, at any event, was my experience.

'At the final stages, too, it is such a comfort to have someone beside you who is not occupied with the physical business of delivering the baby but can concentrate on telling the mother what is happening. That it won't be long now, that there will only be a few more pains, that the baby's head is through, and at the last pain can immediately satisfy the mother's first thought—boy or girl.',

*Mrs D.* 'It is not easy to remember accurately the thoughts and feelings one had some three days afterwards, but this much I do know: that I *don't want* to forget it as most other women seem to; I want to be able to re-live the second stage at any rate and remember the lovely sound of Anne's first cry.

'I refused to believe I was in labour until assured by the nurse about midnight that this really was the real thing. Even so, I never once got worried or felt I couldn't go through without assistance. I didn't change in the second stage either, but just felt confident that everything was going "according to plan." It never occurred to me to have anaesthetics because the contractions just didn't hurt; somehow they seemed to be miraculously converted into something I could conquer myself, and I found great pleasure in the effort involved. I can well understand how painful they could be if you didn't know how to cope with them.'

# APPENDIX

## SOME ADDITION TO THE EXERCISES GIVEN IN THE ANTENATAL CLASSES FOR THOSE CONDUCTING SUCH CLASSES ONLY

(Illustrations have therefore been felt to be unnecessary)

**Pelvic floor static contractions**
Cross-leg lying.
Crook lying. Knees opening out when relaxing.
Prone kneeling.
Kneeling.
Sitting.
Standing, heels and toes together.

**Pelvic floor exercises** *N.B.* The hips are also included to render them more mobile).
Squatting and rising (feet flat).
Lunging.
Walking upstairs two at a time.
Leg swinging in all directions.
Kneel sitting (with glutei on the floor and legs one each side), bouncing up and down gently.
Kneel sitting. Sit first on one side of the feet then on the other.
Crook lying. Placing both knees on the floor, first on one side then on the other.

**Pelvic tilting** *(straight abdominal work)*
Crook lying.
Prone kneeling.
Kneel sitting (sitting first in front of, then behind, the heels).
Squatting.
Kneeling.
Arm lean standing.
Standing or stride standing.

## Abdominal exercises
*Lateral*
  Prone kneeling: hip wagging from side to side.
  Prone kneeling; walking, hands round towards hips.
  Kneeling, sitting, kneel sitting, stride standing; side bending.

*Rotary*
  Prone kneeling. Swing one arm under the body and then out and up to the ceiling, turning to look right up at it.
  Sitting (kneel sitting, stride standing, kneeling, half-kneeling.) Trunk turning.

# BIBLIOGRAPHY

1. Alan C. Beck. *Obstetrical Practice.* Williams & Wilkins Co.
2. Cyril Bibby. *Sex Education: A Guide for Parents, Teachers, and Youth Leaders.* Macmillan & Co. Ltd.
3. Professor F. J. Browne. *Advice to the Expectant Mother on the Care of her Health.* E. & S. Livingstone Ltd.
4. Professor F. J. Browne. *Antenatal and Postnatal Care,* Sixth Edition. J. & A. Churchill Ltd.
5. Marie Campbell. *Folks do get Born.* Rinehart & Co.
6. Professor M. Edwards Davis and Mabel C. Carmon. *De Lee's Obstetrics for Nurses.* W. B. Saunders Co.
7. Wilfred Thomason Grenfell. *Yourself and Your Body.* Hodder & Stoughton.
8. Howard W. Haggard. *Devil's Drugs and Doctors.* Wm. Heinemann Ltd.
9. Edmund Jacobson. *Progressive Relaxation.* University Chicago Press.
10. R. C. Jewesbury. *Mothercraft, Antenatal and Postnatal.* J. & A. Churchill Ltd.
11. L. S. Michaelis. *How the Body Works.* Longmans, Green & Co.
12. Merrel P. Middlemore. *The Nursing Couple.* Hamish Hamilton.
13. Alan Moncrieff. *Infant Feeding.* Edward Arnold & Co.
14. Florence Powdermaker and Louise Grimes. *The Intelligent Parents' Manual.* Wm. Heinemann Ltd.
15. Minnie Randell. *Training for Childbirth.* J. & A. Churchill Ltd.
16. Grantly Dick Read. *Natural Childbirth.* Wm. Heinemann Ltd.
17. Grantly Dick Read. *Revelation of Childbirth.* Wm. Heinemann Ltd.
18. Grantly Dick Read. The correlation of mental and emotional phenomena in normal labour. *Journal of Obstetrics & Gynaecology,* February 1946.
19. Grantly Dick Read. *The Birth of a Child.* Wm. Heinemann Ltd.

20. K. de Schweinitz. *How a Baby is Born.* George Routledge & Co. Ltd.
21. C. F. V. Smout. *The Anatomy of the Female Pelvis.* Edward Arnold & Co.
22. Frances Bruce Strain. *Being Born.* Arthur Barron Ltd.
23. Kathleen Vaughan. *Safe Childbirth.* Bailliere, Tindall & Cox.
24. Kathleen Vaughan. *Childbirth an Athletic Feat.* Reprinted from the *Medical Press and Circular,* 26th December 1945, Vol. ccxiv., No. 5564.
25. Kathleen Vaughan. *The Enlargement of the Pelvis in the Squatting Position.* Reprinted from the *Medical Press and Circular,* 21st March 1934. Bailliere, Tindall & Cox.
26. Harold Waller. *Clinical Studies in Lactation.* Wm. Heinemann Ltd.
27. Margaret Moore White. *Womanhood: A Book for Girl, Wife, and Mother.* Cassell & Co. Ltd.
28. F. Charlotte Nash. *Breast Feeding.* Oxford Medical Publications.
29. Albert Sharman. *From Girlhood to Womanhood.* E. & S. Livingstone.

# INDEX

Figures in italics indicate page on which illustration appears